OF PEOPLE
& PLANTS

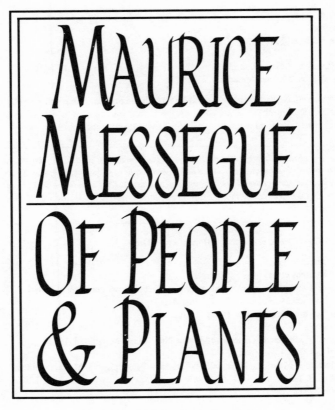

MAURICE MESSÉGUÉ

OF PEOPLE & PLANTS

The Autobiography of
Europe's Most Celebrated Herbal Healer

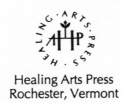

Healing Arts Press
Rochester, Vermont

Healing Arts Press
One Park Street
Rochester, Vermont 05767

First Healing Arts Press edition 1991
Copyright © 1991 Maurice Mességué

Note to the reader: This book is intended as an informational guide. The remedies, approaches, and techniques described herein are meant to supplement, and not to be a substitute for, professional medical care or treatment. They should not be used to treat a serious ailment without prior consultation with a qualified healthcare professional.

LIBRARY OF CONGRESS CATALOGING-IN-PUBLICATION DATA

Mességué, Maurice.
    [Des hommes et des plantes. English]
    Of people and plants : the autobiography of Europe's most celebrated herbal healer / Maurice Mességué. — 1st Healing Arts Press ed.
    Translation of Des hommes et des plantes.
        p. cm.
    Originally published : Of men and plants. New York : Macmillan, 1973.
    ISBN 0-89281-437-3 (pbk.)
    1. Mességué, Maurice. 2. Herbalists—France—Biography. 3. Materia medica, Vegetable. I. Title
    [RS164.M39513 1991]
    615'.321'092—dc20
    [B]   91-26306
                                                                  CIP
Printed and bound in the United States

10 9 8 7 6 5 4 3 2 1

Healing Arts Press is a division of Inner Traditions International, Ltd.

Distributed to the book trade in the United States by American International Distribution Corporation (AIDC)

Distributed to the book trade in Canada by Book Center, Inc., Montreal, Quebec

Distributed to the health food trade in Canada by Alive Books, Toronto and Vancouver

Contents

vi *Contents*

OF PEOPLE
& PLANTS

1

The Plant Expert

BACK HOME we have a saying: "To know a river you have to know its source."

For me, that source was my father, cherished as a well-spring in our native land where water is scarce—a pure, fresh, bubbling spring amidst a profusion of sweet-smelling wild plants. Everything I have I owe to my father: my love of life, whatever I know, whatever I have achieved. He alone shaped the entire course of my life. To understand what this means is also to understand my deep love for him.

I was born on Sunday, December 14, 1921, at 4:30 in the afternoon, under Sagittarius, and by chance at Calayrac-St. Circq (Lot et Garonne)—a little slip-up soon rectified by my parents taking me back, when I was only three days old, to my grandfather's house in Gavarret. My village patriotism is such that I always say I was born in Gavarret in the Gers, firmly pronouncing the final *s*. That is my terrible Southern accent, because of which I love these lines by Miguel Zamacois:

> Avoir l'accent, enfin, c'est chaque fois qu'on cause,
> Parler de son pays en parlant d'autre chose.
>
> To have an accent means, no matter what else on earth
> One talks of, one's talking, too,
> About the dear old country of one's birth.

I even enjoy listening to my own talks on radio or tele-

vision, for those accents make me see the familiar landscape, the country paths, the wild rabbits; feel the stones
beneath my feet, sense the fragrance of our wild herbs.

Sons, grandsons, great-grandsons of country folk, the
Mességués have lived on the same land for over four hundred and fifty years and have always had this special knowledge of plants. I remember being treated with herbs when
I was still a tyke of four or less. I was sleeping badly, tossing
and turning in my one doubled-over sheet, whimpering,
my legs reddened by the rough, coarse linen. The next
morning my father said: "The child isn't getting his sleep,
we'll give him a linden-blossom bath." That evening my
mother set out a big copper basin and my father said:

"Look, my boy, that's copper, it's finer than gold. It's
red like that because it has been a mirror to the sun and
the fire, and you are going to have a bath in it."

Then my mother poured into it a golden liquid she had
been warming and I was plunged into the linden-blossom
bath. I let out some blood-curdling yells, but she kept me
soaking in it up to my neck, and then I remember feeling
very sleepy in the bath and being carried to bed by my
father. I didn't know it at the time, but I had just had my
first lesson.

In those days drug-induced sleep was not the common-
place it is today. Linden blossom was picked all warm in
the sun and buzzing with bees, and spread out on canvas
sheets in the shade.

"The secret," my father would say, "is not to let the plants
die and turn to dust; you have to get all the good out of
them while they still have it."

So when the linden blossoms were barely dry, not bone-
dry, they would be left to soak in huge copper basins full
of water, and the resulting infusion was then stored and
could be used five or six times for bathing a highly strung
child. My father often put me to sleep in this way and I
have done the same for my own sons.

When I delve deep into my memory, I can see the

beams in our big farmhouse kitchen, where bundles of herbs would be hung to dry, heads down, alongside the game. It was a pretty sight, those bouquets of buttercups, greater celandine and poppies alongside the brown hares and the fat red partridges you find in our part of the world. I can still see my mother, so pretty and dainty and full of life opening the cupboard every Saturday to take out one of our two pairs of sheets, fragrant with the big bunches of lavender my father used to bring home in armfuls. She used to change the bed on a Sunday, and when she had finished she would lovingly stroke the sheet with her weather-beaten hand, that busy hand that could do everything, shyly saying: "Your father will like this . . . " She worshipped my father, and to do her justice, he was an unusual man, different from all the men who worked the land thereabouts. He had no land of his own—we were too poor—and he did not even hire himself out as a laborer. He had his own way of loving the earth: he did not till it, but he looked at it. The earth was his book of the knowledge of good and evil. He spent hours studying it, but he didn't actually *do* anything. My maternal grandfather took a poor view of this and grumbled at him, although it might well have been my grandmother who put him up to it. But my grandfathers hardly had any right to talk. They were every bit as peculiar as my father; all of their time was spent arguing. One of them was a partisan of the Republic, the other a Bonapartist, and they would sit and glare at one another for hours, hotly debating their differences of opinion, much to the entertainment of the villagers who would come to listen to them.

My grandfather Edouard was nicknamed "the African" because he had done his military service in Algeria. In those days conscripts were still picked by drawing lots, and he hadn't been able to pay for a substitute. To have in their midst a man who had done his service at Sidi-bel-Abbes was a source of constant amazement to the locals, and they would gather round on the long winter evenings to listen to his tales of black men and Arabs and that beast of the Apocalypse, the camel. It was only a little village in Gascony. Those were the days before there was tarmac on the village street, so it was muddy in winter and dusty in summer. We all wore wooden clogs, our only lighting was from oil lamps, and there weren't even enough lamps to go round. You carried a candle to light you to bed, and thought yourself lucky. Our only heating was a log fire and, like many families, we cooked our soup in a stockpot hanging over the fire.

There had been no shortage of "drones" in our family. One great-great-grandfather had been a schoolmaster round about 1850, which was a step up if you like, but not of any real significance—the only thing that counted was the land and the ownership of land; anything else was merely illusory. Another had gambled and disgraced the family name: he had lost money. It's one thing not to make money, but actually to lose it! He spent the rest of his time hunting. They were nearly all "contemplative" types; it was a family failing, and they were never mentioned when the children were present. When I went to catechism, the curé would fix me with a meaningful look whenever we recited "Laziness is sin," "Idleness is the root of all evil."

Our idleness was a trait we attributed to our ancestors in distant lands, for it was certain that Moorish blood ran in our veins. I myself look like a bandit! I believe and, for the sake of family honor, always maintain that one of my great-grandmothers must have been raped—although for her sake I hope she enjoyed it—at the time of the battle of Poitiers, when we were invaded by the Moors. One day I was having my eyesight tested by an oculist—I, too, sometimes have to consult doctors, specialists in particular. He told me: "The whites of your eyes have a characteristic found only in the Moors." I no longer recall the scientific name he gave it. However, what is certain is that both by taste and inclination I am very much in sympathy with Spain and the south and the sun. Whenever I go to Sweden or

Norway I can't wait to get back, but whenever I go to Spain or Portugal I feel I could stay there forever. When I see the mosques around Granada I feel as if I have been familiar with them for generations, and I think I must have lived with the Moors because I understand them. I understand their passion, their pride—and their carefree attitude towards life.

My father spent his life contemplating, observing, watching—and they called him an idler. Nobody understood how wise a man he was, not even my mother. It was difficult for her, short of money as we always were, to understand why my father worked so little, and often not at all. He was very sensitive about it, with the acute sensitivity characteristic of the Moors. Like the Moors he had a particular fondness for roses, his favorite flowers: "My child, roses are beautiful and full of healing power."

He loved scents too, and around him there was always the clean fragrance of lavender, never the smell of sweat or tobacco or wine. He used to drink a great deal of coffee, and he also drank an unheard-of beverage, mint tea. He kept his powdered mint and tea in big jars and mixed them himself. No one knew how or where he had acquired these tastes. Perhaps from "the African"? I never saw him drink a glass of wine; he was never drunk in his life. People considered him peculiar. They said, with utmost scorn, "Camille drinks water."

In Gavarret he was out of place, like a duck in a hen run. He wasn't cast in the same mold as the rest of the villagers, being small and almost fragile in appearance, and he was further distinguished by his mode of attire, which made him look like a dandy in an English engraving. He dressed much as we do today, in a Cardin-type double-breasted suit with rather high lapels. He wore a tie and shaved every day, his moustache was thin and neatly trimmed and he always used a table napkin! He had only one pair of shoes, but he wore them often, like a real gentleman. His hands were another extraordinary feature, small and soft and young-looking, with slightly stubby fingers, like the hands of a child, and his fingernails were always clean and properly trimmed. You can imagine what our local peasants must have thought of this man, with his clean white hands, every time they passed, shouldering their tools and carrying their hayrick covers and other heavy loads. Moreover, our district was by current standards very leftist —radical Socialist—and my father, poor as he was, inclined very much to the right. Worse, he was a Royalist. It was unthinkable: a peasant in a forgotten village in the Gers—without newspapers, without radio—who was a Royalist! I think that for him it wasn't so much a matter of political opinion as of aesthetic taste. He loved history, and all those kings with their glorious courts and palaces and gardens. Even their wars must have appealed to him more than the *Bonnets rouges* and the smell of cheap wine that characterize the merry-making of the plebs.

If we had lived somewhere else, somewhere less easy-going, all these things might well have caused people to hate him, reject him, treat him as an outcast. But in our part of the country, folk are kindhearted and they mostly considered him mildly odd: "He's a funny fellow, Camille," they would say. He did strange things, like eating oysters. He ate them only once, it is true, but the entire village came to watch: they were beautiful, clean, green oysters he had brought back from the market in Auch, and he opened one and said to me: "Smell that, you can smell the sea." Much later Léon-Paul Fargue remarked when we were lunching together one day: "Whenever I eat oysters I can taste the sea."

For a long time I was almost obsessed with the thought of the sea, until when I was eighteen I went to Arcachon with the rugby team. I was trembling with expectation at the thought of seeing the sea and eating oysters, my very first oysters, but when we arrived the tide was out, and the Arcachon basin allows no view of a distant horizon. As for the oysters, they were small and flat and beige.

2

Animals Know

My FATHER was something of an oddity in the village, but the people respected him. He used to hunt—in fact his nickname was "the hunter"—and he did a little poaching too, an activity that was widely approved in our neck of the woods. He was also a water-diviner, and lastly he used to cure people. I say lastly because we didn't think anything of it. All our family had done the same: my grandfathers *and* grandmothers and even my mother.

My father, with his generosity and total honesty, was easily taken advantage of. If ever he found water or healed someone and my mother said: "Camille, you ought to make them pay you," he would reply: "Nobody makes me pay for water or plants. All I had to do was find them."

People came from three or five miles around to consult my father. When he was dowsing for water he used his hazel wand, for the pendulum was unknown in our district. He taught me how to hold the wand when I was still quite small, and I remember dropping it in fright the first time I felt it move. But I soon learned to accept that a branch could move by itself, and I was proud that it worked for me. Since then I have found that a pendulum will oscillate for nine people out of ten; they are dowsers without knowing it. Of course the professionals say: "We have a gift." It is indisputable that they have a higher degree of sensitivity and that there are good water-diviners and bad ones, and that, as in everything, experience counts for a great deal. But there are also outward and visible signs of the presence of water: the geological configuration of the land, the plants: horsetail, certain kinds of nettle, certain kinds of buttercups. There's nothing supernatural about all that, and in fact my father used to call them the "water-divining plants." He hated scientific names. "The people who gave them those names might know plenty about science, but they don't know much about plants." Years later, when I was up against the Medical Council, I often recalled his words, and they helped me considerably.

As a small child I would see him come home bearing great armfuls of plants, many of them in bloom. Later I would go with him, and he would point out the various herbs and plants.

"My son, see that 'stinging grass' (the nettle), how hairy and rough it is, but if you know how to take hold of it, like that, quite firmly and from below, it won't sting you. When it's cooked it's very kind to the stomach and the digestion."

For him the greater celandine was "the swallow's flower," which for centuries has been called the plant that makes a sick man weep if he's going to die or sing if he's going to get better.

"You can't mistake it; if you break one it will weep great orange tears, and it's good for everything; it's my favorite flower. The rose is the most beautiful, but the celandine is the best." He used to include it in all his preparations. He would also tell me about *Achillea millefolium* (milfoil), which he called "the carpenter's plant": "You see, it's good for healing a cut." Such everyday names helped me to love and know the plants.

He used about forty different plants, but his favorites, the ones he used most often, were: single seed hawthorn, artichoke leaves, buttercup, greater celandine, creeping couch-grass, watercress, corn poppy, common broom, lavender, peppermint, nettles, parsley, dandelion, broad-leaved plantain, blackberry bramble, sage, crimson clover, cabbage rose and sweet violet—twenty or more. Then came: milfoil, garlic, shepherd's purse, spring heath, cabbage, male fern, corn, round-leaved mallow, onion, meadow-sweet, followed by knapweed, borage, great burdock, sweet brier, mistletoe (*viscum album*), juniper berries, bloody burnet and field horsetail.

On the evenings when he said, "There's only a sliver of a moon tonight," this told me that the next day we'd be out gathering plants. "My boy, remember, never when there's a full moon; moonlight saps their strength. For plants to be at their best they need plenty of sunshine and very little moonlight. Meadow sage is at its best cut at dawn on a midsummer morning."

We would set out very early in the morning, our clogs making a nice cheerful clatter as we marched down the road. By ten o'clock the sun was too hot for picking herbs, so we would stop, and my father would produce from his game-bag some bread and garlic and sometimes a bit of goat's cheese, which we would eat slowly, savoring each mouthful as peasants do. Then at about four in the afternoon we would go on gathering more plants until nightfall. Gently, lovingly, my father would snap a few stems, break off some leaves or pull up a root.

"My boy, the goodness of a plant isn't always in the same place. Sometimes it's in the head (the flower), sometimes in the body (the stem), sometimes in the feet (the roots)."

And so I learned that only the berries of the juniper, the petals of the rose, the beard of corn, and only the leaves of plantain are beneficial. It was important to gather the plants in the right season, and in spring and summer we would set out nearly every day. "My son, now is the time when the plants are rich and full of love! But in winter they grow cold and sleepy." In this way the seasons passed and the years went by. No happiness in the world could be great enough to make me forget those days spent with my father.

The first time I saw him heal ànyone it was a neighbor, a man I knew well and whom I saw regularly morning and evening as he passed by. One Monday on his way home he came into our big kitchen bent double: "Camille, d'you think any of your plants might do me some good? I've got a kind of stabbing pain just here," indicating his right side.

"That's your liver."

"You reckon? But I'm not sick."

"You might not be, but your liver is, and it's telling you so."

"In that case I can't say I'm enjoying the conversation."

Whenever people came to my father he tried to make them laugh. It was good for them and took their minds off their sickness, making them more receptive to the goodness of the herbs.

"Camille, give me your treatment here. I don't want my wife to see."

My father took down some bottles from over the fireplace and mixed several liquids in a bowl. He then made a compress by folding a small piece of flannel, soaked it in the liquid and placed it on the man's side. Within half an hour the pains had gone and his face was no longer screwed up out of all recognition as it had been. Gripping the table in my excitement I couldn't take my eyes off him: it was a miracle! "Papa, did *you* do that!"

"Son, he who causes the plants to grow is the one who did it."

My father was a simple man and his fame never traveled farther than a radius of seven miles or so. He didn't see more than five or six persons in three months. Yet he was better known than I realized at the time, as I later discovered. People had heard of him from much farther afield, only they didn't come to see him—anything over ten miles was considered quite a journey. He was mostly consulted for liver disorders, because people drank too much and ate such heavy food, but he also handled cases of congestion of the kidneys, which he treated by getting his patients to urinate. Often they came to him with "pains": "Camille, I've a pain here," "I've a pain there," they would say, tenderly feeling themselves on the arm or the leg or the back. Or "Camille, I can't breathe."

He was successful in his treatment of asthma, which in those days could be traced to simpler causes: allergies are diseases of civilization and progress. Nowadays, air, water and food are polluted by chemicals which we then breathe or swallow. My father used to treat asthma with foot-baths. He would drop what he called his macerations into three or four litres of water, and his patients would soak their feet in this for quite a time. He had learned this from my grandmother, who had learned it from her father and so on, going back generations.

My father had been taught by his father, an extraordinary old man, a giant, consulted even by people who came to him all the way from the city. This was a source of great pride to him, and he would willingly oblige you with an account of these visits. But for a long time now, whenever anyone asked him for treatment he would reply: "Go and see Camille, he knows, I've given him my macerations." He had also given him the family "Plant Bible," which was only a few sheets of paper handed down from some distant ancestor who had scarcely known how to spell and so had made drawings of all the plants he used, alongside a note of their therapeutic virtues. Whenever he was puzzled, my father would take these papers out of the sideboard drawer and mull over them.

Where we lived my father was known as the "Plant expert." When people came to consult him, he would press his ear to their chests and say, "The clock's ticking nicely" (meaning the heart, of course) or, "The clock's out of order." It was all very simple, the kind of thing they could grasp. To go to the doctor was to take a step on the track that might lead to one's death, and to go to the druggist was to board the train that would get one there. If you bought a medicine it meant you were very ill indeed.

The doctor was a person of great importance in our community. He was seldom seen about, so everyone was astonished when it became known that Dr. Lapeyre, our local doctor, had come to my father for treatment. As he did not want it known, he had waited until nightfall, left his gig some distance from the house, and then crept along in the shadow of the walls. My father had been greatly surprised to see him.

"Camille, I'm suffering from fluid retention."

"Retention, Doctor?"

"Yes, my body's retaining fluid. Do you have any plants to make people urinate?"

"Ah, if that's all it is, then I can help."

The house suddenly became a hive of activity. My mother set plenty of water to boil and my father called to me: "Go and get the mint, bring some nettle, don't forget the celandine, the beard of corn and the sage." While I was fetching the plants the doctor was undressing. Finally, stripped of his clothes but not his dignity nor his monacle, there in our kitchen Dr. Lapeyre sat in a hip-bath of my father's plants. He had shed his self-important airs, and behaved just like an ordinary man towards my father, whom he usually treated so patronizingly. Thereafter, as my father's plants had relieved him, whenever the doctor came to make his calls in the village—no oftener than once a month —he always had a moment for my father, and my mother would stand by as he drank a glass of wine.

Yes, Camille could heal, but for him it was a simple act, an act of charity in the theological sense of the word "caritas." I don't think he had "the gift" or that he could mesmerize people. He was interested in the occult, but it was a straightforward interest, a probing into the continuity of man and the benevolent forces of nature. Yet even when

I was quite small I felt that my father had an aura of extraordinary power, that he was a man born out of his time. He was handsome, his eyes were not like the eyes of ordinary mortals but shone with a religious light. Everything about him had a shining quality; he gave such an impression of real power that you had no choice but to submit to it and let it warm your heart and marrow, filling you, washing over you like a great wave of love. I have always thought that he transmitted this power to his plants and that they were somehow enriched by it.

Certainly my own conviction is that there are forces other than those recognized by science and the five senses. I need quote only one very simple psychological example: the saying: Laughter aids the digestion. You can eat a huge stew with your schoolmates and digest it with no bother at all, whereas you can get indigestion eating a leaf of lettuce in boring company.

What most amazed the local people was Camille's way of living. "He seems to have plenty of time," they used to say. I can still see him in my mind's eye lying flat on his belly in the meadows at the edge of the wood, spending hours watching the rabbits and hares, who were not at all afraid of him. I would stand near and he would say: "My son, you don't learn about life by dashing about in every direction. You learn by looking—see, these animals know more about it than we do. They know the plants and grasses, which are good for them and which are bad, they know what to eat and how to take care of themselves." He was right. A wild animal living free never poisons itself, for it knows what foods to choose. This is an instinct animals lose when they are domesticated. A tame rabbit in a hutch can no longer sense the dangers of scarlet pimpernel and will eat it and die; a cat living in a city apartment will eat lily of the valley, which is very harmful to it. Certain dogs, such as alsatians (wolf-hounds), that are still close to their ancestry, distinguish two kinds of grass: the slightly hairy grasses, which they use as an emetic, and couch-grass, which they use as a purgative. A Pyreneean mountain goat with an injured leg has been known to make itself a plaster of clay and grasses, using its mouth. The weasel, before attacking vipers, will roll itself on a plantain, the leaves of which are very effective against bee-stings and viper poison. My inherited love of animals led me to make my own land into a "reserve." I bought this woodland, where my father used to gather plants and which used to belong to the Comte de Lary, both for the plants and in memory of my father.

For me the only good plants are those that grow in the Gers, on my native soil. These plants are my faith, and I believe that if I were ever to be dishonest with myself I would no longer be able to heal. I have been healing for thirty years, and looking back I know that I have never been dishonest with a patient, not even for an instant, and I believe that this matters tremendously. Patients feel that I will make them better, they tell me so and I do not doubt it. That, too, is a legacy from my father.

3

The Death of a Happy Man

MY FATHER was worried about my future. He saw that I
wasn't very robust, that I wasn't built for tilling the soil, and
this made him anxious. With his foreknowledge of things
and people, did he sense that he would quit this earth so
soon?

He was happy with his life; it was a life that suited him,
but he would wonder: "Will my son feel as I do about
the land I love? I live for my plants, but will this be enough
for him?" He knew well enough that there were other things
in the world besides Gavarret and Auch, and perhaps he
had even dreamed of them himself, who knows? He was
fully aware that his kind of indifference about making a
living was not possible for everyone, that his plant lore offered no kind of economic security. Using herbs to heal
people was all very well, but he could not see it as a paying job. No, he was absolutely determined that I should
be a civil servant: someone who was well-dressed, with a
pension and holidays and a respected social position. Such
was his ambition for me. Moreover, he had a particular
kind of civil servant in mind. I was to be a chauffeur at
Police Headquarters in Paris. This had been a cherished
plan for me from my birth, and all because of Paul Jansou.
This Jansou was a fellow who had got on in Paris. Everyone goes there nowadays, but at that time it was quite

something, and he was spoken of for miles around. "He's done all right for himself," people would say. He was our local celebrity—and he was a chauffeur at Police Head-quarters. People practically crossed themselves whenever he spoke, and his word was law in the village. Disputes were held in abeyance until Paul stepped off the train.

Camille would make a point of paying his respects to Paul, thinking that he was working for my future. Each year, when Jansou came home for his month's holiday, he would take him the freshest mushrooms and young partridge shot the same morning, arranged on a bed of vine leaves in a wicker basket covered with a starched white cloth. Then my father would say to him: "Perhaps one day you'll be good enough to recommend the lad . . ." This was almost fifty years ago, but Jansou is still going strong —and the villagers still doff their caps to him.

Meanwhile, to prepare me for such a fine situation, Camille would speak to me in correct French: "My son, dialect is the language of the soil, it came from the soil. But French is the language of your country, the language of towns and educated people, people who 'know.'" It would never have entered his mind that he might "know" more than they. I can still see him as he sat of an evening at the table, reading *Le Chasseur Français* by the light of the oil lamp that always smoked a little. The book was full of stories about animals that he would later tell me, speaking in that gentle, slightly hesitant voice of his, choosing his words carefully. It was with the help of *Le Chasseur Français* that he taught me to read, pointing to the pictures of animals and birds and plants and teaching me their names. He also used to cut out letters and assemble them to form words that I would spell out. I had no alphabet as such, and I wasn't taught to read the way most people are. Nor was I taught to live the way most people do, which is perhaps why I am a happy man.

As soon as I knew how to read and write I was sent to the elementary school in Gavarret. I had an elderly teacher named Drancourt, who still came to school on horseback. One day he fell ill and was replaced by a lady teacher. I thought her terribly pretty, and for the first time in my life I fell in love, only to meet with my first big disappointment, for the postman used to linger to court her. I still smart at the memory! Mademoiselle used to come to school on her bicycle, and I remember her skirts as being very short, although whether they really were I'd no longer like to say. In any event, her legs were very pretty in their fine stockings! I was dreadfully jealous of the postman who, in my eyes, had dark designs on the lady, although I granted him his fine moustache. So I pinched my mother's knitting needles and punctured the postman's tires. I must have made at least a hundred holes in them. That was the one and only time my father ever gave me a hiding, and it made me feel very grown up to think that I had suffered it for the sake of my great love.

By the time I was ten I had learned all I could at the village school, and so I was sent to the lycée in Auch. A town of streets where nothing grew, classrooms as big as our entire house, schoolfellows who were not all sons of country folk—for me it was an amazing adventure.

My first school year passed quickly. But at the end, when I was eleven, my father died in a shooting accident. His gun went off as he jumped over a ditch. When I reached home that evening the house was full of women all in black, mournfully saying their beads, while the men left their clogs outside the door and entered two or three at a time, removing their hats and standing still, embarrassed by their own bulk and their too obvious robust health. They would say a word or two to my mother and my aunt, and then leave. That night I learned that the "queer fish" had been loved.

They told me that my father was dead, that he was lying on his bed in the bedroom for the last time, but I refused to see him and I do not regret it. The last memory I have of my father is not of a dead man on his bed but of the living man who used to call me "My boy." I was filled with grief, but I did not know that my happy times were over for many years to come.

The death of my father was the most terrible thing that has ever happened to me. I have never admired anyone as I did my father. He was a man remarkable in his wisdom, his knowledge. Handsome and distinguished, he seemed to possess every fine quality a man could have, and I worshipped him.

4

"Grey Smock's" Revenge

W<small>HEN I WAS</small> twelve my uncle took me by the hand and marched me off to Lectoure. I was a scholarship boy, starting as a boarder in the Maréchal Lannes school.

It was a warm autumn day such as we get in the Gers, when the sun shines as hotly as in summer, but as soon as I found myself enclosed by the high walls of the schoolyard, I felt suddenly cold. I knew that the light of day would never enter there, that in such a place days would always be grey. I looked at the three dusty trees, prisoners as I was, scapegoats, scarred and stripped of their bark, indescribably sad. Beneath them the earth was hard as stone, beaten down by schoolboy clogs. There wasn't a plant to be seen. How could I possibly live without plants?

And then everything changed: in a cleft in the wall I noticed a sprig of celandine. It was a miserable little specimen, not glossy with good health, like the celandine I knew, but it was celandine none the less, my father's "magic" plant

Nobody has ever used celandine as my father did and as I do now. Externally its juice is used chiefly on warts, as an antiophthalmic, on strumous tumors and on scorbutic and atonic festering ulcers. I include it in all my preparations. My father used to tell me how he had discovered one of the medicinal virtues of this plant when watching a nest of swallows under the eaves: "You see, I saw the mother bring a sprig of celandine to the nest and as it clearly wasn't intended as food for the young ones I wondered why." By patient observation he finally discovered the answer: the swallow was holding the celandine in her beak and rubbing it against the head of one of the fledgelings, always the same one, the one whose eyes were still shut. When his eyes finally opened, the mother bird no longer brought any celandine. The properties of celandine had been noted long before his time, but my father's inspired empiricism had rediscovered them. I can still hear him saying: "Every part of the celandine has its uses—the leaf, the flower, the stem and the root—and it's good for everything." I have also observed that in a preparation it brings out the virtues of the other plants.

For me the celandine is also a lucky charm, and I certainly needed it on my first day at the school in Lectoure, even though I had gone there with plenty of confidence. In my last class at Auch I had won twenty-two prizes, including the prizes for gymnastics and singing. It took me only a few days to grasp that my "laurels" were just a bunch of pathetic, dry leaves that impressed nobody.

Being poor and without a father to stick up for me, I was fully exposed to the natural cruelty of schoolboys and often had a tough time. I was the only one of the boarders who did not have a tuck box in his locker to supplement the terrible school food. The others would eat their home-made sweetmeats and *pâtés* and jams right under my nose, and one of them—today he considers himself a friend of mine —would hold his sausage under my nose and say, "Here, have a sniff, it'll give your bread some taste." Indeed it did—the taste of bitterness. They spared me none of their uncouth jokes: one evening, while I was getting ready for bed, they took my one and only sheet, soaked it in the wash-basin and then put it back on my bed sopping wet. I spent that night shivering on the floor. Every winter I suffered so indescribably from the cold that I would pick up and hoard every newspaper I found to cover myself with at night. Not until I was in the upper fourth, did things improve a little, for by then I was on the school rugby team and so the teachers saw to it that I was given a sheet and lent a blanket.

But what most hurt my Moorish pride was the business of my school smock. I wore the same smock for three years. The first year it was too long, by the third year it was too short and tight—it was splitting at the seams, and it had turned grey. This earned me the nickname of "grey smock," and silly though it was, I was hurt and fought many a desperate fight on account of it.

Nobody made any allowances for me. Apart from the headmaster, the teachers all treated me unkindly. At the least sound, the slightest smothered laugh in class, the teachers didn't even bother to turn around but said: "Right, Mességué, leave the room!" I don't pretend that this was always undeserved, for I was very unruly, probably because I was always being ragged and ridiculed and so I learned to act the clown, to assert myself, to take the lead instead of being a mere victim. They had no reason to concern themselves about me, since they knew that no parent would turn up on Saturday to complain to the Headmaster or threaten to take their business across the road. Across the road was the competition, the free school run by the Abbé Tournier. My mother would never have dared to come and complain. By now she had gone into domestic service and was working nearby as a maid in the house of a banker named Bastide. In order to be near her son she had at one time even worked in the school, which was hard on me and even harder on her. She was the butt of constant cheap jokes; in fact the boys jeered at her so much that she didn't stay long, although long enough for me to be known as "the servant's kid" ever after. I loved and admired my mother, so if I felt humiliated by their gibes, it was only on her account.

The misery of being poor among the sons of well-to-do landowners was more severe on Thursdays and Fridays (market days in Lectoure) when their parents came to take them out, and excruciating on Saturday evening when they'd go home for the weekend, while I was stuck there, as pitiful as the three trees in the yard. On Sundays a teacher would take me for a walk round the town, which clearly bored him to death—doubtless he had better things to do!

I know all the outskirts of Lectoure from having tramped every inch of them in all weathers. These walks, though burdensome to the teacher, used to bring me back to life. I would run along, cape flying and clogs clattering, and—best of all—I would gather plants, despite the frowns of the teacher who found it humiliating to be walking through the town with this ridiculous ragamuffin of a boy who looked like a gypsy and had fistfuls of weeds hanging from his pockets. Before we went back into Lectoure he used to say: "What do you do with all those plants, eat them?"

"No, sir, I just fool around with them."

"Then you'll kindly get rid of them all before we reach the town."

"Yes, sir," I'd say, but there were always a few bits left at the bottom of my pockets, and at night beneath my sheet I would breathe their fragrance and fall asleep with a handful of sage or succory or poppy beneath my cheek. It was only much later that I dared to answer: "My father used them to heal people." Some of the teachers knew that I was the son of "Mességué who treated people with herbs," but I was too small and young for them to think of asking me anything.

A scholarship boy is expected to be the top of his class, but I did not make it because I had to earn my pocket money by doing the other boys' homework for them. I was paid five cents per assignment, ten cents for Latin, and that's how I eventually saved up enough money to buy myself a pair of clogs with leather uppers.

We no longer had a home of our own. My mother lived in other people's houses and I was supposedly in the care of one of my uncles, although he never came to see me and took me into his home only for the long summer holidays. I used to work for him—making hay, cutting corn and tying it in sheaves, in short all the heavy jobs. Not that I minded —I was in the country and that was enough for me. It is still what matters most to me today. Comfort and luxury have made no difference. My idea of perfect happiness is still a hunk of bread, a clove of garlic and a warm hearth. Another thing I liked about being at my uncle's was that I could treat people with my plants: nobody made fun of "Camille's remedies," or of Camille's son, who knew them. At that time there was very little farm machinery in our region; most of the work was still done by hand. The men used bill hooks, scythes, axes—and accidents occurred frequently. As people had no idea of hygiene, wounds very easily became infected. (I remember my father telling an injured man, "Go get some Roquefort from Chicabout [the grocer]" and then making him take it in homeopathic doses.) I would examine their wounds, and whenever one looked unhealthy, I would say, as he had done, "Go to Chicabout." And people listened to me. I'd never have dared to prescribe Roquefort for my schoolmates and even less for the masters, supposing it ever entered their heads to ask my advice. At school I'd have been ashamed of prescribing cheese for a wound; it would have sounded silly, even though I knew how effective it was. When I was a child, I thought it quite miraculous, but today everyone knows the value of the penicillin contained in the mold of Roquefort.

It wasn't only while I was staying at my uncle's that a little of my father's fame rubbed off on me. There was a boy at school, Georges Dutout, who has remained my friend ever since, and who used to take me every two months to spend a day or two with his family in Fleurance. Sometimes we even spent short holidays there, and for me this was a great treat. His parents always made me feel at home, and I had my share of all the special meals that were cooked for him. Here at last was a place where I was once more "young Mességué . . . you know, the son of

Camille who knew so much about plants." My plants were my last link with my father, with my native soil. I went on gathering them, trying to preserve them, drying them in my locker in the dormitory—I didn't have much else to put in it—cramming them into my desk in the classroom, pushing aside my textbooks and notebooks to make room for them.

I had so few friends at school that I had plenty of time to watch and observe the other boys. I studied their state of health and became quite expert at telling from the slightest change in their complexion or their bearing or in the luster of their eyes when they were out of sorts. I would say to myself: He's got an upset stomach; or, he's bilious . . . and then I'd ask them how they were, in order to see if I was right. They might have thought it odd, but they generally told me and I'd mark myself accordingly. I often got eight out of ten, but I never gave myself 10. I was cautious, even then. When I had a mental picture of my "patient" I'd ask myself: What would my father have done?—the question I have most often asked myself throughout my life. Then I would recite the appropriate prescriptions he had taught me; in this way I kept them stored in my memory.

I ransacked the kitchen garbage for bottles which I filled with my "medicines." However, they did not keep for long, as I had no way of boiling the water. I did it only to keep in practice, for my concoctions were unlikely to be used. When they got too old I used to throw them away, though it felt like an act of sacrilege. To preserve my father's knowledge was more important to me than anything they taught me at school. Something told me that I had to remember all I had learned from Camille. Whenever I was feeling particularly miserable I would open my desk and, hidden by the lid, I would shut my eyes and fill my nostrils, my lungs and my head with the wholesome, soothing fragrance of my plants. I would be transported from the classroom, to being with my father in the fields and the woods. Thus occupied one afternoon, I failed to hear a shout: "Messé-gué!"

It was the voice of the Headmaster, Mr. Alleman.

"Mességué, is that yours?"

A classmate kicked me on the shin, I lowered my desk lid and saw the Head pointing at something on the floor. Two yellow snails, striped with black like a zebra, one following the other, were gliding majestically across the grey floor of the classroom, like two Argonaut ships crossing the Aegean. It would have been difficult to claim innocence, for a pretty, shining trail indicated their progress from my desk, and in any case it goes against my grain to lie.

"Get them out of here, and open your desk and get rid of all that rubbish! It isn't even as if you were making a proper collection. Your passion for plants will be your undoing. Leave the room, Mességué!"

That day the Head could have had no suspicion that nearly thirty years later, in 1964, he would be writing me a three-page letter beginning as follows:

My Dear Messegue,
Now that, thanks to your own gifts, you enjoy a fame that is international, may I be permitted to remind you of the time when you were a pupil at the school in Lectoure where I was headmaster, a time when you experienced difficulties and even privations. I know that this will not prevent your showing your generosity . . .

You have not lost your generosity of heart and I am happy to congratulate you for it. Rare are the men today who do not attach a financial value to the charitable act . . .

And the postscript, which I found particularly touching:

I forgot to remind you how jealously you used to hide your plants away in your locker. Many a time I had to punish you for it, for to my mind your studies were suffering on their account. But even then you showed the will to struggle and to succeed . . .

In fact, I was generally considered to be rather strange, especially by the teachers who regularly predicted that I would come to a bad end, for I was a good-for-nothing idler.

By the time I was fourteen my peasant reserve and perseverance had made some slight impression on my teachers, and they began to reflect: He would seem to take after his father. Accordingly they would sometimes ask me for "prescriptions," and although they never actually tried them—for they would never have picked the plants themselves, and I was too shy to offer my own decoctions—they did condescend to ask me: "What would your father have done?" I would feel honored, and impart my secrets, but that was as far as it went. They had no real confidence in me. There was one teacher in particular who questioned me often. He was the history and geography master, a man whose gluttony made him subject to attacks of gout. Typically enough, what he really wanted was some kind of miracle cure that would rid him of his pain without depriving him of his pleasures, and he was ready and eager to believe in anything, provided there was no mention of any kind of diet.

On the days when he entered the classroom with a frown, dragging his leg and wearing a big carpet slipper on his foot, we knew that he was starting an attack, and with a bit of luck—from our point of view—he would soon have to keep to his room. I didn't like the man. Once, when he couldn't remember my name, he called, "Hey, there, Grey Smock!" which made me burn with resentment. And when, the same morning, he had taken me aside after the lesson to say, "I'm in for a bad attack, I can tell. Haven't you got one of your father's mixtures that would do some good?" I replied with some insolence, "No, sir, it's an illness we never get in the country." And there I left him, muttering "Fraud!"—another nickname that stuck, but I didn't care, I'd gotten my revenge for the "Grey Smock." In point of fact I did know a very good preparation based on autumn crocus, roman camomile and burdock that would have relieved his pain.

Outside the classroom windows the sky changed with the seasons, the years passed, and my days of persecution were over. I was one of the big boys, I played school football on Thursday afternoons, and on Sundays I played stand-off half on the town rugby team, almost a professional! They paid me two francs fifty and gave me dinner in a little restaurant in Lectoure. The team manager had obtained permission for me to stay out until nine o'clock, and I was driven back to school in a private car. Now it was my turn to be envied by the others.

I had given up gathering plants along the paths and in the woods. I had so often been told: "Maurice, your father shouldn't have wasted his time playing about with 'herbs,' he'd have done better to earn a living for your mother and yourself." I'd been given so many moral lectures from all and sundry, including my own family, that I'd withdrawn into my shell. I no longer talked about plants and had come to feel almost ashamed of the whole thing, as if it were some kind of fault or weakness. It was my time of denial. It was also a time when I was distracted by girls. In our school, classes were mixed, and we had some good times. In the upper second I had been completely infatuated with a girl of my own age, Simone Barrois. She was quite beautiful and her father was a banker in Agen. I was only thirteen, and I loved her with a tremendous passion. In the upper fifth I dreamt of becoming a doctor for love of a girl, Jeannine Cheminaud, who is now a secondary-school inspector. She was a lovely Eurasian, and from time to time she would let me kiss her, a heady experience indeed! I used to recite poetry to her, send her poems, and do her homework. When she wanted to bestow her highest favor, Jeannine would wash my rugby shirt. We lived purely in a world of sentiment, but it was all quite wonderful, and I have never forgotten her.

5

A Poultice for the Admiral

I TOOK MY FIRST baccalaureate at seventeen—narrowly scraping through, thanks to a 19 out of 20 for Spanish and 18 for French, which gave me a chance to sit the mathematics again in October—and my second "bac" at eighteen. During my last year at school I had given up any idea of becoming a doctor, for we were really too poor, and had decided to take a degree and enter the teaching profession. It seemed as though I might after all acquire the respected status my father had dreamed of.

When war broke out I was nineteen, and due for conscription in 1941. I volunteered in the spring of 1940, little realizing as I signed up that I was also signing the end of a chapter of my life: my youth. After the collapse I found myself without a hero's uniform but wearing once more a "grey smock," and working in the postal censorship at Montauban, under the orders of Commandant Muklautz. I owed my "position" to the jealous vigilance of my rugby club, which had pulled strings to keep me in the vicinity.

The censorship department was on the first floor of the post office, and there were about a dozen of us there, both civilians and servicemen, opening letters with steam over special condensation receivers. The work was a source of great astonishment to me. Peasants seldom write letters, and for my father the arrival of a letter was an important ceremony that entailed quite a ritual: the glass of wine for the postman, the close scrutiny of his name on the envelope —mistakes can happen, and you must never open a letter that isn't addressed to you—and then the blade of the knife carefully inserted to liberate whatever the fates had in store. Finally would come the slow perusal of the letter itself. And here was I opening hundreds and hundreds of letters that weren't even meant for me! It went against my grain to read the first letter I opened; it started with "My love," and I blushed with shame, for I felt as if I were peering through a keyhole. I have always kept professional secrets, but since this was twenty-five years ago I think I can say that many of the letters that passed through our hands were written by well-known artists. They used to go on tour, in unoccupied France, and their mail would be forwarded to their hotels. I opened letters from Nita Raya, Maurice Chevalier, Rina Ketty, Pierre Des, Charles Trenet and many others. I came to know every little thing that ailed them, morally and physically.

I used to read these letters with an unaccountable avidity. I felt that through the words of these people, whether I'd heard of them or not, I would learn something. But what? They were tormented by all kinds of emotions, they worried a great deal, they expressed violent feelings, they complained of various physical discomforts. All this aroused in me a curiosity I couldn't explain. I remember thinking that their very handwriting must mean something—but what? Once, seeing a spidery, distorted handwriting, I thought: "That must be a sick, tired old man." Actually, it was the writing of a boy of twenty who said, "I'm not ill, it's worse than that, I just don't want to go on living." A few days later, the same boy was writing in a firm hand: "Everything's fine, I've just heard from her, I must have been out of my mind." He wasn't far wrong—he had been, briefly. There was nothing really extraordinary about any of this, but to me, inexperienced as I was, it was a revelation. I was very naïve and I'd always had a rather simple view of

life: you eat too much, you drink too much, you don't feel
well which makes you grumpy and irritable. It now occurred to me for the first time that it also worked the other
way around—that a person's emotional or mental state
could influence his health. What a discovery!

Ignorant though I was, I already believed in keeping a
careful check on my suppositions. Each time I read a letter that contained phrases such as, "You haven't written to
me . . ." "I don't know what's the matter with me . . ."
"I don't feel well . . ." "I have a headache" . . . "I'm
feeling bilious . . ." I would examine it closely and make
a mental note of the sender's name so that I could subsequently check whether his physical symptoms subsided or
worsened and whether they appeared to originate in the
body or in the mind. I was sure that it was of paramount
importance to calm the sufferer, to help him relax, give him
confidence, understand him: would I have the power to
do this with the help of my plants? I did not formulate the
question outright, but I behaved as if it were the very crux
of my life. Though I was never closer to giving up the idea
of becoming a healer than in the years 1940–43, and
would have looked askance at anyone who might have told
me that I was hard at work on the foundations of my
therapy, I was constantly studying, making notes, tirelessly
modifying my observations and adding to them. Though
my methods were sometimes puerile, I was rediscovering
for myself the principle I was to apply for the rest of my
life: Treat the patient rather than the disease.

All in all, I was being remarkably inconsistent. My mind
was made up to give up healing as a career, and yet it kept
dwelling on the health of persons I did not know except
through their correspondence, and never stopped collecting
plants on my country walks, drying them, making preparations for the treatment of liver ailments, rheumatism, kid-
ney disorders. Though I knew no one who was likely to
ask for my medicines, I justified my illogical carryings on
to myself on the grounds that it was well to be ready in case

someone needed them! But no one knew about me except the Commandant, who had been told, I believe, by the captain of my rugby team some such thing as: "Remarkable fellow, Mességué—his father taught him how to cure people with herbs."

It must have been some such comment that led to my treating Admiral Darlan. He had come to Montauban on an official tour of inspection, and happened to mention to the Commandant that he was suffering from arthritis in the shoulder. It is a type of complaint that often fails to respond to conventional medical treatment. The Commandant then told him he had a man in the censorship office whose father had been known to perform herbal cures—and would he like to give the son a try?

When I was ordered to treat the Admiral François Darlan, former Commander-in-Chief of the Navy, currently the second most important man in all of France, the man whom people called the Heir Apparent—I was stunned. My appointment was for eight o'clock in the morning. By six o'clock I was already standing in line at the market—it was war time, remember—and I was lucky to have obtained, by seven, a cabbage, a bunch of watercress, and an egg!

With my cabbage and watercress wrapped in newspaper under my arm, the egg and a bottle of my solution for rheumatism in my pocket, I presented myself to Admiral Darlan. He was short, on the stout side, and noticeably tense, pacing restlessly up and down the room.

"So you're Mességué. Where are you from?"

"From Gavarret in the Gers, sir."

"We're from the same parts. I'm from Nérac, not far away."

Not a bit flustered, I found myself taking an instant liking to him. I had no notion of worldly power, and in the presence of this unassuming man, my awareness of his exalted rank had become so purely theoretical that I remained serenely unimpressed and even forgot to address him as I had been told to, calling him "sir" instead of "Admiral"!

He was simply a man in politics, and that such men made history had not yet registered with me. Besides, I was preoccupied with the fact that this was my first real patient, and was busily making mental notes: high-strung, florid complexion, out of condition for lack of exercise—like one of my schoolteachers who ate too fast and gave himself indigestion. The Admiral's eyes were clear and sparkling, but I noticed he had drooping eyelids. It was not what you could call a diagnosis, but it was a start.

"So you treat people?"

"No, my father taught me a few treatments that help in certain cases."

"Well at least you're not a fibber. What do you prescribe: drops, infusions?"

"No, for your trouble I make poultices with plants."

"All right, get on with it then! It's my right shoulder that's bad."

I could see that he was in a good deal of pain. He had difficulty taking off his jacket and shirt—and no one dared help him—and then he sat in his vest saying, "Go ahead!" I was temporarily taken aback at the sight of the froth of grey hairs on his chest above his white vest, for although I had previously given prescriptions, I had never in my life actually treated or touched a patient or applied a poultice.

"What are you waiting for?"

"I need a bowl and a fork to beat the white of an egg."

With that I thought he was on the point of getting dressed again.

"It's some old wives' remedy you're giving me, is it? Ah well, somebody fetch him what he wants, only get on with it, I haven't got all day."

I chopped the best leaves of my cabbage fairly fine (discarding the thick ribs), along with the watercress and some stinging nettle, and bound it all together with the stiffly beaten egg white. Then I spread the preparation on to some muslin, forming a kind of poultice, folding it and pouring over it about a teaspoonful of my maceration, which was based on meadow-sweet, common broom, roman camomile, clary, great burdock, single seed hawthorn, creeping couch-grass.

While I was preparing the poultice Darlan kept questioning me: "What's this for? Why are you adding that?" and I found it hard to explain because I hardly knew the answers myself, being largely content to do as my father had done. He also wanted to know what was in my bottle.

"Do you use plants that other people don't know about?"

"No, sir, I don't think so. The difference is in the way they are combined. My father, too, used to mix plants said to be for internal use only with those to be used externally."

I applied the poultice to his shoulder, telling him: "You must keep it on all night."

"And that's all?"

"No, the treatment also includes hand-baths."

He smiled, almost laughed out loud.

"You intend to make me take hand-baths?"

"They're essential. You have to take one in the morning before breakfast, and one in the evening before dinner. I'll leave my bottle with you."

"Do you really believe in all this?"

"Yes, sir."

Had I been asked the same question an hour before, I'm not sure how I would have answered, but certainly not as I had done now, with absolute conviction. The force of my own "yes" astonished me, and it was enough to convince the Admiral to take his hand-baths. I realized then that my own confidence in myself counted as much if not more than the patient's confidence in me.

Luckily, Darlan didn't ask me the reason for these hand-baths, for I wouldn't have been able to tell him. My father used to prescribe them, so I did likewise. How he learned that the palms of the hands and the souls of the feet are especially sensitive and receptive, I do not know, but the knowledge certainly went a long way back, part of the oral tradition handed down in our family. As I learned later on, the Romans had used their thermal waters in the same way, and at Royat, above Clermont-Ferrand, foot-baths were the prescribed treatment for arthritis. The curative powers of treatments by osmosis are now scientifically explained and accepted.

The Admiral's readiness to believe took me by surprise; I had yet to learn that a sick man who has tried everything is ready to accept anything at all, even—perhaps especially —something he cannot understand. The farther away you get from traditional medicine, which has been unable to help him, the readier he is to believe. Far from being put off by mystery, he finds it reassuring; hence the success of so many quacks.

My encounter with Darlan changed nothing in the pleasant, lulling sameness of my life. Every Sunday I played football for the Montauban team, every month I was paid what would now amount to three dollars for opening letters that weren't addressed to me. The sun shone, the girls were pretty and they seemed to like me, and I asked for nothing more. I felt a sudden stab of uneasiness when the Commandant sent for me and said: "Mességué, you're to leave tomorrow for Vichy. Admiral Darlan has asked for you. He says you made him a lot better and he wants to see you again. Don't forget to take your 'herbs'!"

I didn't much like the idea.

"Will I be away for long, Colonel?"

"For three days, the regulation time for a consultation."

I filled my suitcase with plants, not forgetting my solution for rheumatism, and set off, excited to see the new capital of France. It was a long journey from Montauban to Vichy, but an official car was waiting for me at the station, flag furled. The chauffeur, in naval uniform, was a little chap about my own age who spoke with an accent as thick as mine, which put us on good terms immediately. He had me sized up at a glance for the country bumpkin that I was.

"Ever been to Vichy before?"

"No, it's my first visit."

So like a good pal he told me that in Vichy there were more inhabitants to the square yard than in the most over-populated city in the world: "And be very careful, ears are sharper than microphones. And not so reliable. If they don't like the look of you, you can lose your job from one day to the next! You can't trust your own shadow, the police are everywhere, in uniform, in civvies, city police, state police, the Marshal's police, Darlan's police, the Secret Police, Intelligence Department police, German police—you name it. Everyone's spying on everyone, if not on his own behalf then on somebody else's. They even go through your wastepaper basket like scavengers. It's as good as a promotion to them if they can inform on you. To listen to them you'd think they all had influence. The lowest orderly in the Ministry hotels will try to get something out of you, telling you he can help you, he's pals with the secretary who's the cousin of the typist who works for Doctor Méné-trel,[1] who can whisper in the old man's ear. Which is a joke all right, because the Marshal's deaf! I don't know what you're here for, but be on your guard."

I said nothing, this being as good a time as any to guard my professional secret, as I would have done in any case.

"They're putting you up at the Hôtel du Parc. That's pretty unusual, they only put the top brass there as a rule. You must have plenty of influence."

I had to let him think so.

Walking a bit stiffly in my best suit—to my mind a very fine garment, though the ersatz wool (the wood, that is) of which it was made had begun to crack alarmingly at the elbows and knees—I walked in the hotel entrance hall complete with cardboard suitcase and all the artlessness of my twenty years. My first time in such a palace! In the dining-room I sat at a table laid with silver, half of which I'd no idea how to use. A squadron of waiters, led by the

[1] Doctor Ménétrel, Marshal Pétain's doctor, was reputedly the power behind the throne.

maître d'hôtel, stood ready to serve the guest of Admiral Darlan. I handed over my ration coupons, which must have surprised them, and calmly worked my way through a banquet that was a far cry from my usual "fixed price" meal at The Golden Pheasant in Montauban.

In Vichy, Darlan struck me as more on edge than the first time, worried, at times even snappish. This time he was not alone in the room; there were several men with him, secretaries probably.

"Gentlemen, let me introduce my wonder worker. He must be a bit of a magician, this boy—I'd hardly been able to move my shoulder for three years and now it hardly hurts at all."

He'd thought of everything: a cabbage, a bunch of watercress and an egg. I felt like a conjuror, having to perform in front of such an audience.

"And come and see me again in the morning before you leave. I expect I'll have some news for you."

His news was surprising, to say the least.

"I've told the Marshal about you and he says next time you come you're to give him your treatment too."

At Montauban Darlan had questioned me at length about "rejuvenating" plants. He'd asked if I knew them, if I believed in them, if they were able to increase the vitality of a man in good health but getting on in years, what effect they might have on his sight and his hearing. As a result of this conversation he had got it into his head I might be able to improve Pétain's deafness.

"So you're on your way up, my boy, but don't let it give you a swelled head."

There was no danger of that, I was so totally guileless and uncalculating. But that day I learned that the one thing people don't mind giving away is the name of their doctor or their healer. In fact they'll even go out of their way to tell you, for everyone likes to think his doctor is the best.

Back in Montauban I never mentioned Darlan or the

Marshal, for fear I would be taken for a braggart. Besides, I never really believed that I would get to treat Pétain, and I was right.

The next time Darlan summoned me to Vichy, he seemed disillusioned, almost bitter. He greeted me with his customary "Ah, there you are, my little wonder worker!" But his heart wasn't in it. He had no one with him, unlike the last time.

"Are you happy in Montauban?"

"Oh, yes, sir."

I gave this extra emphasis, in case he had some notion of keeping me there with him.

"Well, that's a good thing, it's certainly easier for you to be happy than it is for me. By the way, I've raised your monthly pay to two thousand francs. Don't thank me, I'd have liked to do more. But it's all off with the Marshal—he mentioned it to Ménétrel, who won't allow it." He shrugged his shoulders. "Perhaps it's as well, after all: it's better the Marshal doesn't hear too clearly what people are saying about him. Here you are, here's your fee."

And he gave me ten thousand francs. A fortune! I took it to be a gesture of kindness the Admiral wanted to make to a fellow countryman, for I couldn't really believe I was being paid for my plants. My father had never had a penny from his patients, who were content to leave a few eggs or some butter or a duckling on the corner of the table, and not always that.

"My shoulder's giving me no trouble at all, but leave me a bottle of your mixture, just to be on the safe side."

I left the bottle and took my leave. My stay had lasted twenty-four hours, and my career as "healer and wonder worker" to the Vichy Government was over. I never saw Admiral Darlan again. He had been my first real patient, and his assassination in 1942 really shook me.

Once again I was breathing the steam in the censorship department. Time passed, we were in 1944, and I was one

of the contingent designated for STO.[1] When I failed to
turn up one morning, some policemen came for me.

"Get your bag, you're leaving!"

Along with some others I had been sent for by the Germans, who considered me a troublemaker, someone who
went around undermining the German war effort by advising Frenchmen not to go to Germany to work for those
brutes, who weren't going to last much longer anyway.
There were lots of us on the station platform, and we could
hardly have seemed like enthusiastic "volunteers," since our
little flock was guarded by the police and surrounded by
the militia. I didn't exactly love the Germans, but I positively loathed the militia. When they told us to board the
train, I climbed in one side and went straight out again on
the other. Just like that, and it worked. After that there
was no way out for me other than to join the maquis.[2] I
linked up with the Tarn-et-Garonne group and they gave
me a little aluminum Cross of Lorraine bearing the number
145. My group was part of the secret army of the Dordogne,
and at the liberation I fought in the Pointe-de-Grave, the
famous "Royen pocket" northwest of Bordeaux.

Once I was demobilized I rejoined my mother, but I
couldn't stay with her for long. I was twenty-four years old
and it was time I started making a living.

[1] *Service du Travail Obligatoire* (Forced Working Parties).
[2] Guerrillas who fought in France for the Liberation.

6

A Healer in Spite of Myself

IN SEPTEMBER 1945 I managed to get a post as assistant-master supervising prep in the Fénelon school in Bergerac (Dordogne). It wasn't much of a job, but I was thankful for it. Besides, what else could I do?

It was a few days before term started. I had rented a room, not much bigger than a monk's cell and not much better furnished either, but it suited me. My window looked out over the rooftops of Bergerac, their round tiles glowing in the sunshine with every shade of orange and crimson; a pleasing sight needed to restore me, for I had just been to visit Fénelon. It seemed a bleak enough institution, and the Headmaster, Mr. Decotte, even bleaker. He was a cold man with an icy stare, and his very skin seemed lifeless: I saw at once that he must have stomach trouble, probably some kind of acidity—milfoil and some garlic and round-leaved mallow would do him good—but I had to put a stop to this kind of reflection once and for all. I had decided I would no longer allow myself to think in terms of healing.

With these thoughts turning over in my mind, I felt the bitter taste of melancholy. How vast the sky was above the town—and how small my own future looked. I had given up the idea of taking a degree, I no longer hoped for any-thing, I no longer even dared to cherish any ambitions. Of course I would have liked to succeed—but at what?

The first morning I went for a walk in the nearby countryside. As usual I gathered plants, along the pathways, on the grassy slopes, in the hedgerows: buttercups, greater celandine, peppermint, nettles, sage. This was more than force of habit, it was a need, the one thing that kept the bond between my father and me alive. As long as I continued to do this I was keeping him alive, as it were, or giving him another life. Thanks to these expeditions, my little room was filled with plants. I hung them up, I spread them out all over the place, they lay steeping in the washbowl and in jars. And as of old I started filling glass bottles, bottling my dream . . . There in my room at least I was at home, and nobody could make me throw away my herbs. When I opened my door and smelled their familiar, wholesome fragrance I felt good.

At this time I wasn't actually miserable, only torpid. My future looked like a dead end, to be sure, but this did not prevent me from living intensely in the present. Life in itself was a marvelous thing, after all, and happiness is a state of mind. I am lucky in having a natural aptitude for it. Even on my worst days, a tender blade of new grass in the morning dew has always filled me with such profound joy that I have wanted to thank the Good Lord. I don't mind putting it on record that I'm a believer, although not a practicing Catholic. I never go to Mass—there are too many people for my liking. But often when I'm out walking I push open the creaky door of one of those little country churches, and this is where I feel close to God, my God and nobody else's! I kneel and talk to Him quietly, and He listens to me like our village curé, who knew everything about me, the good and the bad.

I was eight years old when our curé taught me a lesson I'll never forget. Being at that age filled with dreams of perfection, I asked him:

"I want to dedicate myself, devote my life to the service of others and become a great Saint. How do I start?"

"It's quite simple, Maurice. You start by going home and

being very obedient and paying attention to everything your parents tell you."

"Every day or just on Sundays?"

"My child, goodness isn't only for Sundays. We must try to be good every day."

It came to me later that with happiness it's much the same: you have to make the effort every day to deserve it. This predisposition to be happy is of such importance that in many patients the lack of it actually retards their recovery. Whenever I'm confronted with the kind of patient who could be called a hypochondriac, I know that the treatment will be longer than usual and the outcome uncertain. Such, very likely, was the case with our Principal, Mr. Decotte. He was a sour, unsmiling individual who thought of nothing but his duty, which he performed with a kind of gloomy relish. On his lips the word "duty" became as grim as a northern mine-shaft. Luckily for me, I rarely came in contact with the great Head himself.

The other teachers at the school took no notice of me; I wasn't considered one of them. The only human warmth, so indispensable to every man, that I was shown was by the lads in the rugby team. That this sport has played such a big part in my life is due to the fact that these men have always given me what I have so often been denied by others. As for my pupils, I let them know right from the start that I wasn't going to put up with any nonsense. I was strict, but I think they were fond of me. Our relationship was based on simple things: I played rugby with them and I cured their ailments.

One Monday at the four o'clock prep period I found one of my youngsters doubled up, with pale face and pinched lips.

"Aren't you feeling well?"

"No, sir, I've got a pain here." He pointed to his liver.

At six o'clock I applied a poultice which he kept on all night, and by the next morning the pain had gone completely. Like all boarders they were poorly fed, and so on

Saturdays, when they went home, they would stuff themselves with sweetmeats, *pâtés,* sausages and stuffed chicken —all delicious but rich and hard to digest. By Monday their overworked livers were acting up, and the less tough would be ill and come to me.

If they had been my only "patients" it would have been fine. But when they next saw their parents they'd say: "I was ill last Monday, but the young assistant-master made me better. I thought he was a bit soft in the head"—making the appropriate gesture—"when he put a poultice of plants on me! I only kept it on to please him, but the next day I was cured. The pain had gone completely." This was how it came about that the following Saturday I would be waylaid in the school visiting-room by the aunt who had "pains," the uncle with stomach trouble, the grandfather who was bent double. At first it didn't cause any trouble, but finally things reached the point where every day the visiting-room was full of people waiting to see me who weren't even parents of pupils at the school. I would see them in the corridor and discreetly slip them their little bottles of macerations and give them a few words of advice.

My notoriety kept within bounds, but people believed in me, and word was getting around. Soon I was seeing more than fifteen people a week, which I thought quite impressive. My father had never seen half as many. But neither had the Principal! About 9:30 that Monday morning Mr. Decotte entered my classroom, looking more sour and disagreeable than ever. By now I was used to him and his unbelievably aggressive manner, but this time he was actually white with rage.

"I wish to speak to you, Mességué, I wish to speak to you im-me-diat-ely," he snapped, dragging me off to his study.

"What's the matter, Headmaster?"

"What's been going on in this establishment is the matter, and a serious matter at that." After more than twenty years I can still see his tight-lipped, hard expression and hear his curt tone of voice. "Yes, a very serious matter indeed. Because of you I am disgraced. I have been made ridiculous before everyone. Yesterday at mass, the Sub-Prefect did not greet me. For the first time, d'you hear? The first time! I asked my wife to go and ask his wife the reason for this public snub—and you know what she answered? 'Do you realize that you have a charlatan on your staff' —you, Mességué—'who uses the school for exploiting the pupils' parents! He gives them medical treatment on State premises! It's scandalous!' What do you have to say for yourself?"

"Nothing."

"In that case you either give me your word of honor never to do it again, or else you leave."

I left . . .

I left because I had had enough of such petty narrow-mindedness. I had given my help to people who had asked me for help, without taking a penny for it. And for this I was being fired. I felt outraged.

In my little room full of herbs, bathed and refreshed, I lay stretched out on my bed, soothed by the good clean fragrance of my plants and recalling, I don't know why, a scene from my childhood. It was at Lectoure one Thursday when we were out for a walk. Our noisy file of schoolboys, all wearing clogs, came to a halt and gathered round a gypsy woman who was selling coin purses, pencils, and the like. The other boys pushed forward to buy something while I stood apart, envying them. It was my first year at the school; I was penniless and keenly felt it! So I was astonished when the gypsy left the others and came over to me.

"Give me your hand, child."

"But I have no money."

"I don't want to sell you anything, give me your hand."

The memory was so deeply buried that I thought it forgotten, yet that evening I could see my ink-stained, rather dirty little paw in the gypsy's thin hand, and I could hear her voice:

"You see, they don't play with you, they leave you out of it. Well! You'll do things they'll never do, and what you do will make you richer than they are. But you'll have to give a great deal of yourself to the unfortunate!"

And she had left me there, still holding out my hand. I was ashamed, sure that she had just been making fun of me, but throughout the rest of our walk I had been unable to put the encounter out of my mind. Why, I wondered, had she said nothing to the other boys with their fine clothes and smart clogs? Some of them even wore watches! It would be easy enough to predict that they'd be rich, they already were. Perhaps, I concluded, she had simply felt sorry for me—and I was ashamed of being the cause of anyone's pity.

In my dormitory I had lulled myself to sleep in a curious way, by thinking of my grandfather's watch (my father didn't own one). It was a large, gold watch that chimed on the hour with a pretty tinkling sound: tinn! . . . tinn! . . . My grandfather would hold it to my ear and I would listen fascinated . . . filled with wonder . . .

That evening in Bergerac I thought I could hear it again . . . Were my memories of the gypsy's words and my grandfather's watch trying to tell me something?

7

Making a Start

Mʏ ꜰᴀᴛʜᴇʀ used to say, "Pride is the poor man's nobility."

I didn't go to make my apologies to Decotte, but decided to set off for Nice. I had picked on Nice because it was the only town where I knew someone, in this case, a Dr. Echernier. He had formerly lived on the outskirts of Toulouse, and in those days he had been my father's "influential friend." He would come by car once or twice a year to see Camille, and bring us sausages or chickens or a ham, which pleased my mother no end. My father would invite him to stay for dinner and, as usual, my mother stayed on her feet to serve the men.

Dr. Echernier, in the course of the meal, often questioned my father about the medicinal value of plants: "Tell me, Camille, what do you reckon sage is good for? We doctors use it especially as an anti-perspirant." And I would see my father nod his head, not daring to say that such words were all gibberish to him. With his Latin subtlety he would reply: "That's very clever, Doctor. I use it to treat people who complain of stomach trouble. But there's more than one kind of sage—I know of three. There's the 'sage of the ruins,' [1] which also thrives in gardens. It keeps well and its powers are long-lasting. Some say you should gather it on

[1] *Officinalis* sage.

45

a midsummer morning when it's at the height of its strength. It's a good tonic, but a bit strong to be taken every day. Then it's better to choose the 'goodly sage.'[2] You find it along lanes and in hedgerows. It's so mild you can take it for a long time, it never sets up any irritation. I don't care for the 'sage of the fields.'[3] It's like certain women, not as good as it looks. It soon loses its scent and its virtues too."

"Camille, d'you reckon a plant isn't any use once it's lost its scent?"

"Ah, yes, when herbs smell of dust it's because to dust they've returned."

My father wouldn't say much more than that. He thought Dr. Echernier knew far more than he did, and he did not care to make a fool of himself.

Dr. Echernier would leave at about four o'clock. The noise of his car would momentarily shatter the quiet of Gavarret, and then everything would return to normal. Camille was rather proud of these visits, not to say vain.

I might have forgotten Doctor Echernier had my mother not received a letter from him during the war. The letter said something like "I am settled in Nice and here it's hard to get food, there is a shortage of everything. If you could send me a little parcel it would be a great help and enable me to bear these restrictions." My mother was very poor, she was in domestic service, but she did what she could.

I had kept the doctor's address in Nice: 3 rue Chauvin. He was a friend of my father's and a doctor, two good reasons for going to ask his advice. I had made my decision; it was as if something had clicked into place inside me and I knew at last what I wanted, what I had to do: I had to heal. My father had healed. He was always a bit surprised at the sort of power his herbs gave him. "They certainly do a lot of good," he would mutter to himself with thought-

[2] Clary.
[3] Meadow sage.

ful satisfaction. But it never occurred to him that there could be a way of earning a living.

That evening in Bergerac I quietly assessed my chances of becoming a healer. Medical school was out of my reach, to my lasting regret. But would it have taught me more about plants than I already knew? Probably not. The Mességués empiricism, founded on generations of practical experience, had proved itself time and time again and I could be in no doubt as to the excellent record of my father's treatments. And now my faith in my own abilities had received a powerful impetus; first, by my success in curing Admiral Darlan. I, a nobody, had been received and treated with respect by a man of importance. He had encouraged me and helped me to overcome my shyness. It was he who first made me aware of my possibilities. Second, here in Bergerac, each week more and more people had been coming to me, because I had done them good and they had told one another so. Word-of-mouth obviously worked: if one cured one's patient, the rest came of itself. For me, it was not a question of making any fortune, far from it; I needed to continue my father's way of life. The problem was, how to make it self-supporting. I lay thinking far into the night: my requirements were modest, my ambitions equally so. I would leave it to the doctors to make the diagnosis, and then simply put my knowledge of herbs and their curative powers at their disposal. Doctors had the scientific knowledge and I knew some good remedies, so we should be able to collaborate.

Later I had to learn the hard way how pitifully naïve, indeed utopian, my thinking was, but that night my ideas were my Evening Star, and that star was leading me to Nice. And so I resolutely shut the door of my "herb" room next day and set off.

I caught the four o'clock bus to Marmande, and there I waited for the seven o'clock train. I was so impatient that every time the train stopped during the night I would get up and go out into the corridor. I can still smell the brass rail I leaned on and hear the tap-tap-tap of the train mingling with the drumming of the blood in my veins; the lights of strange towns were like constellations showing me the way. That night I had a feeling of being master of my own destiny.

By morning we were there. To emerge from the station and see the sunshine and the flowers and the palm trees of Nice for the first time was overwhelming—here, I felt, was the city of happiness itself. I was twenty-four years old and in my wallet I carried all my savings: five carefully folded one-thousand-franc notes.

Without even looking for a room, I made by way—carrying my suitcase—to 3 rue Chauvin. On a handsome white marble plaque was inscribed: "Massena Clinic. Doctor Echernier." It seemed to me the height of elegance to have your name inscribed in marble and I fully expected to find my father's friend installed in princely splendor. It was a shock to find him, instead, in a filthy, dark office, with piles of dusty books and pharmaceutical samples lying about. He looked old and tired.

He didn't recognize me, naturally enough as he hadn't seen me for fifteen years! When I told him who I was, he exclaimed: "Ah! So you're Camille's boy. Ah! Well now, what can I do for you?"

His cold assumption that I had come to ask for something might have put me off, but I told him everything, all about Lectoure and Montauban and Bergerac, and it did me good, for this was the first time I'd ever spoken frankly to another man. He was older than my own father, he was a doctor, he would understand, and so I ended in a rush by confessing my ambition. "So that's how it is, I'd like to treat people. I thought you might be able to send me some patients."

"You must be out of your mind! Camille's son is a madman! Treat people when you're not a doctor!"

"Nor was my father, but he did it."

"That was in Gavarret. He was known, there he was respected. I'm not saying he didn't do some good with his foot-baths, but really, it's all a bit childish, that kind of thing! They'd just laugh at you here, you and your herbs. There are more doctors to the square yard in Nice than any other town in France—and you hope to set up in competition, you, without even a diploma to your name? There's no limit to what they think they can do where you come from! [4] What did you say your name was?"

"Maurice."

"Well, Maurice, I haven't much money"—that much was apparent—"but here are fifty francs. Take my advice: catch the next train back and make your apologies to your Headmaster. That's the best thing you can do. One day you'll thank me."

"No. Thank you, Doctor. Well, if you won't help me, it's too bad. I'll manage somehow."

"You'll be sorry. Nice is a jungle."

But my mind was made up, and his kind of thinking, no matter how sensible, could not stop me then, nor have all the obstacles and struggles and the mean, tough opposition ever since turned me from the direction in which my father's life pointed me: "The man who spends his life being of service to others has earned his own," he used to say. This was his philosophy, and I had made it mine.

Dr. Echernier had proved a disappointment and his warnings had fallen on deaf ears, because I did not realize that I was proposing to practice medicine illegally. I had never even heard of the Medical Council and the associations, and the vast, powerful apparatus that existed to protect organized medicine against incursions from outsiders. We were to get to know one another before very long, however. For the time being, it was a glorious day in sunny Nice. Heady with hopes and brimming with plans, I was the classic Young Man from the Provinces come to challenge the Big City: Nice, here's to us both! The first thing was to

---

[4] The Gascogne is to France somewhat as Texas is to the U.S.A. It is the home of the expansive temperament and the tall tale, the "Gasconade."

find lodgings suitable for receiving patients. I installed myself at a pavement table at the Ruhl, my suitcase at my
feet, drinking a coffee and scanning the ads in *Nice-Matin*
for a lodging. The orchestra played, the people were smartly
dressed—I was glimpsing the luxury life at last! For the
price of my one coffee in Nice I could have bought a good
meal in Bergerac. But that day nothing was too good for
me!

In this happy frame of mind, I went to see a furnished
room at 5 avenue Durante. It was on the eighth floor and
there was no lift, but there was a kitchen and all the usual
facilities. The landlady turned out to be from Bergerac; her
familiar accent at once put me at my ease. I told her I had
just left her home town.

"Ah, you were at Fénelon school! Well, then, in that
case it's all settled, you can have the room."

She was looking me over, even so, and her inspection
proved expensive: "Where's your luggage?"

I pointed to my suitcase: "There."

Whereupon she claimed, quite untruthfully, that in Nice
it was customary to pay six months in advance, and in a
wink had extracted 1200 francs from my tiny hoard. I realized that my youth and my dented cardboard suitcase did
not inspire much faith in her, and could only congratulate
myself that she didn't know that my entire fortune was
on my back: a shirt, a pullover and a suit. Probably I also
had a pair of socks and two or three handkerchiefs and
maybe a spare pair of trousers, although I wouldn't swear
to it.

When I put the huge, old-fashioned key in my pocket
and felt it, so cold to my thigh but so warming to my heart,
I was filled with a happiness out of all proportion to the
realities of my situation. My lodgings were of the humblest,
but I was thrilled with my room at the top of the house,
with its little balcony where pigeons came and ate from my
hand, and the tiny kitchen, not much more than a cupboard, but with running hot water. What luxury!

I had only about 3800 francs left, so there was no time
to waste. I found a printer to make some cards: "Maurice
Mességué. Herbal Treatments. Hours 2–4 P.M." I stuck one
on my door with a drawing pin and stood back to admire
the effect. Magnificent! A vision of a brass nameplate crossed
my mind, but I rejected it as an extravagance—and felt
that I was being wonderfully sensible. All that remained
was to inform the *concierge* of my plans. I gave her one of
my cards and told her: "When people ask for me, show
them the way up and be sure to give them clear directions
so they don't get lost."

"Will there be a lot of them?"

"Certainly, quite a few every day."

She clearly thought I was mad, and she was right.
Wrapped up in my dream, I hadn't stopped to consider that
there were no passers-by to see a card stuck on a door on
the eighth floor of a building at the end of the corridor on
the right. Moreover, I had neither friend nor relation to ad-
vertise my services, no one to send me even one patient.

But such niggling considerations could not enter a mind
filled with the satisfactions of leading the ideal life at last!
Every morning at dawn I set out on foot to collect my
plants in the countryside. Above Cimiez and towards Mont
Agel I would gather thyme, the like of which I'd never
seen before, far stronger than our local thyme at home. Then
I would go towards the petit Febron, where sage and greater
celandine grew in profusion, or to Les Baumettes and La
Lanterne, and along the river Loup, where I would gather
buttercups and meadow-sweet.

The plants around Nice are remarkable, perhaps not as
good as the plants in the Gers, but decidedly superior to
the plants I have since tried to grow in the country round
Paris. I selected and gathered them with meticulous care,
leaving any that were too puny or too mature and would
soon have finished flowering. I loved handling plants: more
than fourteen years had gone by, but my father's hand still
guided my own. Everywhere I walked there were red roses

—my father's favorites, the kind I always placed on his grave every All Saints' Day—cascading over walls, pouring out of every garden, suspended from every balcony like the hangings for some perpetual Corpus Christi procession.

At ten o'clock exactly I would sit down under an olive tree and eat some bread, a clove of garlic, some sausage or some goat's milk cheese, and drink some water. It was blissful. This was a period of preparation of learning, of discovering plants that were new to me, such as rosemary, savory, fennel and marjoram. To learn what I could about them, I had bought some books from a little bookshop near the lycée: Maiclef's *Atlas of French Plants*, Cazin's *Treatise on Indigenous Medicinal Plants*, Perrot's work on the same subject, and Roques' book on the common plants. While these books did not add much to my practical knowledge of healing, they increased my learning. I could now set up in practice, reassured that my ancestors had known nearly everything needful about curative herbs and the art of using them.

I would settle myself down on the balcony to read, but always listening for a knock at my door, as I still thought people would come and consult me. I spread out my plants, I hung them on the balcony and in the kitchen, I steeped them, I made up my preparations and poured them into bottles, which I then labelled. My chemist's shop was ready; I had plenty of plants—but no patients. Not a single one. Time was passing and my money was melting away, until I had hardly any money left at all.

That was when I decided to carry suitcases. I had no idea that to be a luggage porter you had to be a union member. To get the general idea, I hung about at the station and learned that the smart train, the train with the well-lined wallets and handbags, was the "Train Bleu." Accordingly I went to meet it and shouldered suitcases from the station to waiting cars and nearby hotels. To be a freelance porter is not an altogether enviable situation. People paid me what they felt like paying, which wasn't much. But it was too much as far as the other porters were concerned, the union members who wore a cap and a metal number hanging like a medal on their jackets, who resented me and called me a blackleg who was taking the bread out of their children's mouths. They had the law, the regulations, on their side and had me thrown out. Someone had told me to "try the big hotels, that's where the money is," so I did, and I got more than I bargained for. I had the entire staff on my back—bell-boys, carters, porters, the lot. It seemed I was cheating them of their tips and my presence lowered the tone of the hotel. The hall-porter at the Négresco even went so far as to call me a "no-good, down-at-heel beggar, a tramp and a scoundrel." He also swore that he'd "kick me up the backside" if he ever caught me setting foot inside "his" hotel again. I don't know which of us would have been the more astonished had we been told that I would be back some day—as a guest. In the meantime I was left without any means of earning my daily bread.

8

I Pay My First Patient

IT WAS WHILE I was carrying suitcases for a living—and a meager living it was—that I often passed "Schoum the Tramp," a professional beggar who operated beneath the railway bridge between Avenue de la Victoire and Avenue Masséna. The bridge forms a kind of long tunnel, dark as a cave even at the height of summer, damp, dirty, smelling of urine, full of draughts and constantly shaken by the trains passing overhead. It was a kind of beggar's court full of tramps, beggars, panhandlers, and hawkers—a whole population of crawling, obsequious vermin presided over by Schoum. He didn't beg, he merely waited for what was his due.

He was a skinny, filthy fellow about fifty years old, with a very long beard and a big hat. Everyone knew Schoum; he was one of the picturesque sights of the town and people gave generously to him. Begging in Nice is a profitable occupation: Schoum grew so rich that he was murdered five or six years ago, beneath the very bridge where coin by coin he had amassed a fortune.

I fell into the habit of greeting him each time I passed, probably attracted by an air of dignity that set him apart from the others. I went so far as to ask him: "Why do they call you 'Schoum'?" "It's on account of my bottle," he told me. A bottle of red wine stuck out of one of his pockets, and a bottle of "Schoum" [1] out of the other. Drinking was the nearest thing he had to a regular occupation, and when his liver rebelled, he swallowed some Schoum to help the wine along. He was a man of experience, remarkable poise and self-assurance. When he got to his feet and left his tunnel he always knew where to go for a meal. I didn't. And so, after the hall-porter at the Négresco had given me the boot, I went to Schoum.

"Mr. Schoum," I said, "it's like this, I don't know where to get a meal."

He raised the brim of his dirty felt hat, scratched his head, looked hard at me and said: "Follow me."

That was how I found myself in the soup kitchen, sitting opposite Schoum. I never knew where he came from or anything about his background, for he never talked about it, but what struck me was that he said "damnation!" like a gentleman. He was covered with dry eczema; it was all over his hands and his face and he would scratch himself even while he ate, his scabs falling all over the place. The sight revolted me, and so I asked him: "Would you like me to treat your eczema, Mr. Schoum?"

He didn't even deign to look up, but went on scratching and eating as if I hadn't said a word.

"Mr. Schoum, would you like me to treat your eczema?"

This time he looked at me, and in his rather cold blue eyes I could read what he was thinking: Who does he think he is to interfere, this seedy-looking individual who carries suitcases!

"Listen, boy, I sleep at the poorhouse every night and let me tell you, the sisters there have tried everything. They've daubed me with blue and red and purple . . . man, they've put me through the whole routine! I'm stuck with my eczema for life, we'll die together. And you've got the gall to talk about treating me! Are you a doctor? No. So dry up!"

[1] A popular remedy for biliousness.

The next day I had another go at him: "Mr. Schoum, wouldn't you like me to treat your eczema?"

"Get lost, kid!"

The third day I had an inspiration.

"Mr. Schoum, if I give you a bottle of wine, will you come and drink it at my place?"

"Why?'

"So I can start your treatment."

"What?" He always said "what?" when he didn't know what else to say.

"Every time you come I'll give you a bottle of wine."

"All right then, I'll give it a try."

It wasn't just because he was such a nauseating sight that I was so determined to treat Schoum; his tenacious eczema was a challenge.

That morning towards the end of November '45 I had risen at dawn. To this day, I get up and go to bed with the sun, like the chickens. After nine o'clock I start yawning, and it's an effort for me to go out or do any work in the evening. My campaign strategy against Schoum's eczema was spread out over the table in the form of little heaps of herbs, and I felt them to check whether they were dry enough and fresh enough. My hand is so sensitive that it beats all your hygrometers; it never makes a mistake. Greater celandine, for example, must be used when semi-fresh, and this is vitally important. Its roots, like the roots of couch-grass, should still be soft, its stems never completely brittle, and its flowers should still retain their fragrance.

I rubbed the driest herbs between my hands, and went back and forth to the kitchen to look over my macerations, some of which I had prepared the day before, modifying the amounts, adding a pinch here, extracting a pinch there. I wasn't preparing a treatment for just any old eczema but for Schoum's eczema. My success depended on the ingredients being combined in the correct proportions, and somehow I felt my whole future depended upon this success.

After giving Schoum's case much thought, I decided to

focus my treatment on his liver and bowels, to rid them of all poisons; his kidneys, to stimulate them to eliminate the toxins in his body; his nerves, to subdue the itching; and his skin, to treat the scaly patches of eczema.

For his liver I relied mainly on the artichoke, not using the flower, which is the edible part, but the unusual and beautiful grey leaves, the acanthus leaves of our vegetable gardens. Country dwellers used to treat jaundice most successfully with the roots of "artichoke." It helps to promote the flow of bile, the elimination of water, and of urea in the blood. As it will also cure certain skin infections of hepatic origin, it was the miracle plant for Schoum. I supplemented it with milfoil, cabbage leaf and thyme.

For his intestines I chose the charming, humble white hedge bindweed, such a modest little plant that it often goes unnoticed, but nevertheless an excellent purgative. My father used to warn me against chewing the stalks, and I have cautioned my children the same way.

For Schoum's nerves I chose linden blossoms and single seed hawthorn, the lovely "whitethorn" called by Binet "the valerian of the heart." It is one of the best anti-spasmodics in existence, having none of the toxic effects of those chemical tranquilizers so freely indulged in today.

As a diuretic I used common broom—held in high repute since 1701 when it rid the Marshal of Saxony of a dropsy that had defied the most skillful doctors of the day—and the flowers of meadow-sweet and the roots of couch-grass.

Lastly, to treat the skin condition itself, I chose sage flowers and the leaf of great burdock, which my father used to call "scurf grass" and of which I use mostly the roots. This plant is considered one of the specific remedies for scaly and impetiginous eczema. I also included greater celandine, which is at once diuretic, purgative, cholagogue (for the bile) and narcotic, and is successfully employed against ulcers and scurfy affections.

This selection of plants represented no new discovery on my part. I was only doing what my father had done, although no longer so blindly: I was beginning to work out the reasons for his choices. At the time I could not have discoursed so learnedly and with such precise medical terminology regarding my treatment for Schoum. It took me years to accumulate this sort of knowledge, and the concomitant self-assurance and authority. I probably owe my self-confidence in part to my appearances in court, for in order to defend myself I was obliged to keep a tally of my cures— over fifty thousand! Such a figure is enough to make even the most timorous man presume a little, and entitles him to speak from experience.

At last I was ready. I even had Schoum's bottle of wine on the table, the bribe I had to pay my first client in that most unusual city, Nice. I don't think I have ever been so nervous and anxious waiting for a patient as I was that day, and yet I felt quite confident, rather like some young general about to start the battle that would decide his future. As it turned out, my victory over Schoum's eczema did indeed alter the course of my life.

Getting Schoum to take a foot-bath was quite a challenge; his first concern when he arrived was his bottle of red wine. Inexpensive as it was, it still had to be paid for; so, after taking two foot-baths daily for a month, my patient had lost his eczema—and I my money, to the last dime. But this didn't spoil my satisfaction in contemplating Schoum's beautiful, smooth new skin. On Christmas Eve he said: "Kid, you're a bit of a kook with your herbs and all, and you look a sorrier sight than I do, but you're a good lad so I'm going to take you out for a meal. We'll have midnight supper at the Salvation Army. I'm no sectarian. When the good Lord provides you with food, you don't want to worry about where it comes from!"

And so I enjoyed my sardines and my chicken, without being revolted by the sight of Schoum. I watched him eat with a special affection—for being such a shining success of a patient, I suppose.

Years later, memory took me back to that Salvation Army Christmas dinner and Schoum telling me:

"You know, kid, Mother Marie, the Mother Superior at the Cimiez poorhouse, was thrilled when she saw I'd got rid of all my scabs and my skin as pink as a new-born babe! She asked me how I'd managed it and I told her, 'There's a fellow that goes to the soup kitchen with me, a young chap, it was he who cured me by making me take foot-baths. What d'you think of that, Mother!'

"You know, she wouldn't believe me. I had to show her my feet, how clean they were, and then she knew I was telling the truth. And so then she said you must be very clever to have got such good results and she asked me for your address. She's riddled with rheumatism, poor woman. Tough luck for you: from tramp to convent. You'll never get rich that way—just one kind of beggar after another!"

And Schoum broke into a hoarse laugh, quite unconcerned that his wide-open mouth displayed a large number of black gaps.

9

A Lucky Encounter

AFTER CHRISTMAS I received a visit from Mother Marie. She was about fifty, with a lovely face beneath the winged coif, and obviously an active woman in spite of being considerably on the plump side.

She was the first client to knock at my door. I almost wanted to thank her, but it was she who thanked me for seeing her. I was in a state of great nervous excitement, I had no idea how to set about it. Up to now I'd only given advice, never a proper "consultation." How should I begin? I didn't know that patients are always very "knowledgeable" about their case and that all you need do is to say seriously and sympathetically, "Tell me all about it," and they will. My confused: "How are you, Mother?" luckily accomplished the same thing, for she started at once telling me all about her pains. As I listened I was looking at her thoughtfully. Obviously her spine had to carry a considerable weight, and my first question came quite spontaneously: "Do you have any pain in your legs?"

"Yes, I have a lot of trouble getting about." She looked at me attentively. In the space of a few minutes I had learned that you must first let the patient talk, and then show him that you are familiar with his ailment.

During all the months of waiting, I had had plenty of time to realize that lack of confidence would be my problem and to prepare myself in some way for this first consultation. I had decided that it would help me to control my nervousness and to concentrate if I used the pendulum, an instrument with which I was familiar. Mine was a very cheap and simple affair, an ordinary plumb-line such as draftsmen use. As it happened, it served the purpose very well—and it has gone on doing so for twenty years!

Showing as much delicacy as I could, I examined Mother Marie with my pendulum to check her painful "spots," and at the same time considered what would be the best treatment. My father had treated "pains" with a maceration that included:

Cabbage, that chubby round plant that's sturdy as a peasant. Pliny the Elder declared that the Romans owed it to cabbage that they had done without doctors for six centuries! Cabbage leaf, quickly heated by an iron and applied directly to the skin, will effectively soothe rheumatic pains. In Holland up to a few years ago they used to make an ointment of cabbage mixed with clay, which brought relief when applied to painful spots.

Lavender, thyme and sage, in conjunction with *Roman camomile,* which is well known as a stomachic, but too often ignored for its anti-spasmodic qualities, which act as a relaxant in acute attacks of rheumatism.

In Mother Marie's case it was very important that she should lose some weight, so I had to increase considerably the proportional amounts of diuretic plants. I concentrated on *meadow-sweet,* which would do double duty: Dr. H. Leclerc[1] and Dr. F. Decaux said it had given good results in cases of acute rheumatoïd arthritis; and Professor G. Parturier[2] in cases of cellulitis.

Common broom, couch-grass, and field horsetail, which my father called "Fox's brush" and which has been used

[1] *Précis de Phytotérapie.* Masson, 1954.
[2] Professor of chemistry. Author of *Comment guérir par les plantes (Healing with Plants),* authoritative book on phytotherapy.

successfully by doctors since the sixteenth century in cases of dropsy. And lastly, of course, *greater celandine.*

When Mother Marie left, I went out on to my balcony and whispered fervently "Father, I only hope I'm not wrong."

As it happened, the treatment was a great success. Mother Marie lost more than twenty-two pounds (10 kilos) in fifteen days, and I told her that she looked like a girl again. She truly did, and my compliment made her blush a little in the shadow of her winged coif.

The sisters of her order were nurses who attended people in their own homes. Whenever a patient failed to respond to their treatment, they would say: "You ought to go and see Mr. Mességué, he made our Mother Superior lose weight and he cured her pains." I had acquired more than just a guardian angel—I had an entire convent on my side! By now I would hear someone knocking at my door as often as four times in a week, then twelve . . . Schoum's eczema had changed my whole life, and I was transported with joy!

In the morning I gathered my plants, in the afternoon I saw patients, and in the evening I prepared my macerations. People paid me what they wanted; I didn't dare ask for money or quote a fee. There were some who took advantage and gave me nothing at all or just a handshake, but even so there were weeks when I made as much as two hundred francs—a fortune!

One afternoon a grey-haired plump little woman, Hortense Davo, came to see me. She had thrown a coat over her white overall.

"Mother Marie told me to come and see you. She says you cured her rheumatics and I've got the same trouble, and it makes life very hard. You see, I'm a laundress. So my hands are always in the damp, what with the steam from the irons and all. There are days when I think I can't go on, my hand won't be able to hold the iron. So if you can do anything for me you'd be doing a great kindness, sir. My hand's my living . . ."

I gave her the same treatment as Mother Marie, omitting the field horsetail and the meadow-sweet—there was absolutely no need to emphasize the diuretics. Her legs were bad from so much standing, so I added some stinging nettle, milfoil and broad-leaved plantain, which my father used to call "rats' tails."

"How much do I owe you, sir?"

"Nothing."

"But I can pay," her hand was still in her overall pocket where she doubtless kept her purse, which I imagined to be of solid black leather like the purses of my peasant women in the Gers.

"I know, but you can pay me when I've made you better."

They say a good deed never goes unrewarded, and Mrs. Davo proved a case in point. Fifteen days after her visit she sent a lady to me. I had had no experience of "society," but I saw that this lady was different from my usual clients. Her clothes were of that expensively simple cut that I later learned to appreciate, and on her left hand she wore a diamond. I'd never seen one before, but I knew at once that it was the real thing. She certainly suffered from rheumatism: the joints of her fingers were already knotty and her fingernails bore the telltale vertical lines.

"Sir, I'm the wife of Doctor Camaret. My husband is president of the Menton Medical Association. I told him how much good your treatment has done Mrs. Davo, and he advised me to come and see you."

She spoke quite simply, as if it were the most natural thing in the world for a doctor to acknowledge my existence. For a moment or two I nearly lost my head. I had asked Mrs. Camaret to take a seat, and now I looked at her, wondering what I should do. Should I use my pendulum? Wouldn't she think my questions rather childish? Living with a doctor, she probably knew far more than I did of medical terminology and the like. Would I be making a fool of myself? Then I suddenly had a mental picture of my father treating Dr. Lapeyre. Camille had handled himself full of aplomb, in fact with a certain roguish playfulness attesting to his self-assurance. After all, my words were just as good as any scientific jargon. I calmed down and passed my pendulum over Mrs. Camaret's pretty suit. I then examined her hands, which showed signs of rheumatism similar to those of Hortense Davo's, though they were less deformed by it. Carefully I mixed my preparation for her rheumatism, wrote out my "prescription" for her. Each morning before breakfast, soak the hands for eight minutes, each evening before dinner, foot-baths for eight minutes, which should be taken as hot as possible. I noted that the contents of the bottle I was giving her should be poured into three litres of boiled water, and subsequently reheated but never brought to the boiling point. Then I accompanied my patient to the door, and returned to sit at my desk. I was beginning to believe in the possibility of success; and yet, if Dr. Camaret's wife failed to show any improvement it would be the end of everything.

From that moment it all happened very quickly. Soon I had come to be in pretty general demand, and my room at 5 avenue Durante was beginning to seem very small. Dr. Camaret arranged with the Menton Tourist Information Bureau to put at my disposal an empty villa on the outskirts of town, at the foot of the mountain. I gave consultations there every other day, for by now I had no shortage of patients; quite the contrary, since the Camarets and their friends whom I had treated were sending me new patients every day.

I would catch one of the first buses of the day and arrive in Menton when the town was still sleeping, but already there would be people waiting for me. I never turned anyone away, not because of the money—for more than a third of my patients didn't pay, their treatment was so simple that I didn't have the heart to demand a fee—but because of my own hunger to cure people and my own thirst for experience. I spent at least half an hour on each consultation, which meant that every evening, some went home without having seen me. I was, in fact, accepting too many patients, and especially too many different ailments, not knowing that there were some that I was powerless to help. For me each patient was a profound challenge, so it was hard to turn one away; but I did learn to say "no" when a case was beyond my scope.

Meanwhile the actual collecting of my plants was posing quite a problem. I was the only one who could do it, just as I was the only one who could give the consultations. I often had to ask patients to call back for their bottle of maceration, for my meager stocks were soon exhausted. All this meant that I was living under pressure, and it was at that time that I first met Dr. Camaret himself. I had once shyly said to his wife that I would be grateful for the opportunity to express my thanks to her husband, should he be able to spare me a few minutes. But from the way she had replied, with a polite little smile, "Of course, I'll tell him," I had known that the time was not yet ripe. I waited, longing to speak to him, having so many things to say, and becoming increasingly uneasy with doubts as time went on when, at long last, Mrs. Camaret invited me to their house.

Two days before I was due to go, as I ran to catch my early-morning bus, I caught sight of my reflection in a shop window. Impossible! I couldn't go to the Camarets looking like that. I had never given much thought to clothes before, but what I suddenly saw stopped me cold! It wasn't only that my trousers and jacket did not match—when I wore a jacket—but that I was altogether too color-happy: blue, yellow, red, green, the more the better, had apparently been my attitude. (It seems that I was merely ahead of my time in this respect, but in the forties, such clothes on a professional healer in a conservative, well-to-do French city were rather too far-out for anyone's tolerance.) I hastened down to the old quarter of the town where I generally bought my shoes, because they were cheaper there than in the center of town. But that day I went straight to a real tailor's and bought a suit—the color of pale rose-

wood! It must have been a disaster, but the way I understood it, in my fashion naiveté, was that dark suits were
worn on occasions of mourning only, so I certainly could
not wear anything so gloomy to Dr. Camaret's.

Two days later, at 7:00 P.M. exactly, I rang the doorbell. I was shown into the drawing-room, and while I waited
I rehearsed my thank-you speech. There were so many
things I wanted to say: that I was touched by his confidence
in me, that I owed him everything, that his wife had been
wonderful to me, that . . . And there he was: a man of
fifty, going grey, with a strong and resolute jaw and a
forthright look about his eyes, and a mouth as gentle and
good as the mouth of an apostle in a religious picture.

"Doctor, you have placed such confidence in me that I
would like to thank you . . . no, more than that! . . . without you . . ."

And I told him everything—all about my doubts and
discouragements and my fear of failure. It was the second
time I had unburdened myself to a doctor, but Dr. Camaret
wasn't like Dr. Echernier. He didn't tell me to pack up and
go home; on the contrary:

"I have only done my duty as a member of my profession. I know the medicinal importance of plants and the
extent to which they can aid the doctor. It is too often
overlooked that in our pharmacopoeia there are certain
plants that have never been supplanted: boldu, digitalis,
belladonna, monkshood aconite—and many more. You
possess knowledge we only touch on during our years of
medicine. To me you are a specialist, and I am convinced
that your collaboration can be very useful."

Here was a doctor telling me that what I had always
believed in my loneliness was true: that it *was* possible for
me to work with a doctor.

Each time he sent me a patient I noted down my observations, the composition of my macerations and the dosages prescribed, and improvements or setbacks in the patient's condition, and sent these notes to him so that he

could keep a check on them. It was an extraordinary time of faith and enthusiasm, work and study.

It was then that I came to treat my first celebrity: Mistinguett.

10

My Lucky Star: Mistinguett

MY PATIENTS came from all walks of life, although I saw comparatively little of the ordinary working classes, for I wasn't thought to have "the gift," and mostly they believe either in what they can't explain at all or in science. On the other hand, I was often consulted by the professional classes. These are the intellectuals, the people who feel the need to get "back to nature," who do not blindly admire progress for the sake of progress. They're afraid that science is overreaching itself and they often stop and wonder: Where is the world heading? What are we playing at?

And then there were, of course, the country people, who came to me because plants were something they understood and trusted as part of their daily lives. With all this I had every inclination to be content. I even took special delight in the fact that it was a derelict who had brought me good fortune. And then, quite unexpectedly, my first celebrity came along—Mistinguett, the star who brought me fame.

At this time she had already made several farewell appearances. Even I knew as much, although as a rule I was ignorant of such matters. For me she was the greatest star of them all, the symbol of a world I would never know. I had heard that she had "retired" and was living as a permanent guest at the Hotel des Anglais in Menton, which belonged to her niece, Mrs. Desboutin. That was as much as

I knew, and there was no reason to suppose I would ever know more.

One day a friend of the ever-helpful Dr. Camaret said to me: "You could be just the man for someone I know. Mistinguett."

"You must be joking! She could hardly need me."

"She very well might. You see, it's not her age that prevents her from skipping about the stage: she's crippled with rheumatism. The more I think about it, the more I'm convinced it would be a good idea for you both, only she's a wary woman and she'll want to see you for herself. She doesn't take long to make up her mind, but she won't trust anyone else's judgment."

As he was due to see her the next day, he suggested: "Ring me while I'm with her, and if she's in a good mood I'll get her to have a word with you."

I made the call, although certain that nothing would come of it.

"I'm glad you rang, I was just telling my visitor about your miracle cures. She's having a bit of trouble with her rheumatism and she'd like to see you. I'll put her on."

And then I heard the voice I knew only on records, the voice of Paris-Gavroche: "Hello. They tell me you're good at curing people. Would you try to do something for me?"

I was so overcome at actually hearing that celebrated voice that I stammered and stuttered: "Madame . . . of course, I . . . I admire you so . . . I hardly know what to say . . ."

She burst into that inimitable peal of almost strident laughter, the laugh of Mistinguett.

"Come and see me the day after tomorrow at eleven. And for both our sakes, be sure you don't lose your touch before you get here!"

Me, the kid in clogs from Gavarret, the "charlatan of Lectoure," the "quack schoolmaster" of Bergerac, me, the buddy of the tramp in Nice—I was to treat Mistinguett! Today, I cannot hope to convey what this meant, for she already belongs to another age. But then she was still a very big name, particularly on the coast.

By five-thirty in the morning I was waiting for the flower market to open. I had planned to take her some red roses. The air was mild, dawn was breaking and the street lights along the Rue St. Vincent de Paul were growing dim. On the pavement were great banks of carnations, and behind them were the flower-sellers, calling out in their local accents, bidding one another good morning, exchanging news. The entire street was filled with flowers as if for some great carnival. I looked at the red roses, my favorites, but then I decided that I'd look pretty silly arriving with an armful of roses.

I had nearly six hours to wait, so I took the tram and then walked around the outskirts of Menton. On my way I couldn't resist picking one very simple red rose, the kind I like best, sturdy and beautiful, although I knew I'd never dare give it to her. To wear it in the buttonhole of my smart striped suit would have been even more ridiculous, so I put it in my jacket pocket. Still the schoolboy of Lectoure hiding his herbs in his pocket!

By the time I gave my name at the hotel reception desk I thought I was prepared to meet Mistinguett. The hotel garden was well-tended, fragrant with lavender and roses, with bougainvillaea climbing in profusion among the palm trees, and it was in this setting that she opened a French window on to a terrace. I was standing three steps below, and she made her entrance in true music-hall style, wearing a wrap edged with swansdown and looking as if she had just stepped out of the Casino de Paris. She was exactly as I had imagined her. Flinging wide her arms she called: "Come, young man!"

To me she was more beautiful than an eighteen-year-old. I was so overcome that I didn't think how old she might be—sixty, maybe eighty—but for me, beauty has nothing to do with age. As long as a woman arouses desire she remains beautiful, and Mistinguett is probably the most overwhelmingly desirable woman I have met in all my life. She had tremendous sex appeal—and she certainly knew how to use it. What a woman! I was still stunned as I followed her into her bedroom.

"You use a pendulum, I believe."

In a second she had taken off her wrap and was lying face down on the bed.

"Well, let's get on with it!"

It was the first time I had examined a patient who was nearly naked—the part that was covered was no bigger than my hand. My kind of preliminary examination of the patient does not require that "the patient" undress. I whipped the pendulum out of my pocket with such haste that the rose fell on to the bed. I don't know whether the rapid oscillations of the pendulum were caused by the magnetism of my patient or the trembling of my own hand, but the string with its cheap little leaden weight was powerfully affected as it swung above the kidneys of this millionairess. So was I. She had kept on her stockings and a tiny garter belt—it was a tantalizing sight. What legs! They must have been insured for several million, but no matter how crazy the amount, they were beyond price.

She turned her head to look at me, and in her humble, anxious eyes, I read the eternal question of the sick: "Is there anything you can do?" I became professional at once.

"What are you going to give me?"

"A poultice to apply in the region of the kidneys. You must keep it on all night and apply a fresh one in the morning. I'll make one up for you this evening."

"Don't you keep any already prepared?"

"I can't, because I vary the prescription to suit the patient."

"I'm not surprised. You look serious, too serious perhaps . . ."

I heard her laughing again, and looking down, I saw my red rose on the bed. I reached out to pick it up, but she noticed my movement.

"Did you bring it?"

"I picked it . . . and . . ."

"For me?"

"Yes!"

"How lovely, you picked a rose for me! I shouldn't at all have liked you to buy one—I don't like people who waste money. But we'll talk about that another time."

I was to learn a lot from Mistinguett. "Are some of them pretty, the plants you're going to put on my back? No, you don't have to tell me now, you can tell me after they've done some good." Actually, I was considering how much more cabbage her prescription would require, but I never told her. It was too unpoetic.

It cost me a heroic effort to wait four days before calling her:

"I am much better. Come and see me again."

I went to our second appointment in a state of emotion not much different from the first. Except for Admiral Darlan, this was the first time I had been close to anyone famous, anyone whose work and talent had taken them to the top. I have never believed that anyone can be a success for nothing. With bluffing and clever publicity a person might stay at the top for two, three, five years—but not a lifetime. This was a woman who had worked her way up from nowhere. She had also had famous, rich, aristocratic lovers; men had ruined themselves on her account. To a young fellow from the backwoods she was a dazzling personnage.

She was waiting for me, smiling, and greeted me with: "My little Mességué, the pain in my legs has gone."

She lifted her skirts high, really very high—up to her thighs. The gesture that had made her a fortune, that day earned her only my admiration, my great admiration, and it was as if she were singing just for me:

> *On dit que j'ai de belles gambettes,*
> *C'est vrai!*

> *They say I have a pretty pair of legs,*
> *And so I have.*

She loved showing off her legs, for she knew just how beautiful and alluring they were. Nobody who saw them could forget them, so long and perfectly formed, so tantalizing in their silk: the famous legs of Mistinguett.

"Well then, Maurice?"

From the way she dwelt on the name, I knew she was thinking of that Maurice with the straw hat, the Maurice she had really loved.

"I can tell by your accent that you're from the south, but what kind of Maurice are you?"

"A peasant from the Gers."

"I'm more used to city people, but I'm always willing to learn."

What a menace she must have been, this woman.

"If you hadn't cured me with your plants, you could have tried curing me with your eyes; you could hypnotize people."

"So can you, only you do it with your legs."

"Maurice, I like you. Come and sit here and we'll have a little chat. You seem to be a steady young man."

"I live like a monk."

"Really?" She was making me blush.

"I mean, I eat very simply and I don't drink at all."

"That's very sensible of you. Then I won't offer you a drink."

This little matter of hospitality having been thus settled, she continued:

"Maurice Chevalier and I were virtually ambassadors for France wherever we went—but all that was a long time ago. I've learned a lot of things in my life, things that went in here (touching her forehead) and stayed in. My kind of experience is worth a great deal."

I had no idea what she was driving at, but I listened intently.

"Any ordinary woman would have given you a cigarette case or a fat check. And then good-day, good-night, finish. But me, I'm going to educate you; I'm going to give you advice worth its weight in gold and you'll be able to turn it into gold for the rest of your life. The reason I've told you about Chevalier is because he owed a lot to me. A lot more than he thought and certainly a lot more than he's ever admitted. Let's not talk about it any more. Luckily I'm rich enough and to spare."

These words were unexpected, coming from her lips. I still didn't know her well, but I was beginning to understand her.

"Anyway that's how I'm going to pay you and one day you'll thank me. In the meantime, what's the next stage of the treatment?"

"Foot-baths. You will take . . ." and I set forth in great detail the treatment she was to follow. I went to see her daily, although I was already seeing about thirty patients a day. But for me Mistinguett was special, I had never dreamt of getting within hailing distance, let alone treating her. And here I was, telling her to take foot-baths! One day she said to me:

"Listen, love, you've made me much better, I have far less pain now. Tomorrow you're going to have dinner with me."

I went to pick her up as she had asked.

"Always on time, that's what I like. We'll take a taxi and we'll dine at the Négresco."

There was no shortage of fashionable places on the coast, so why did it have to be the Négresco? Perhaps the hall-porter will see me paying off Mistinguett's taxi, I thought. That should impress him. Or perhaps there'll be a new porter by now. As we got out of the taxi I saw at once that there had been no changes; I knew them all. But perhaps they wouldn't recognize me in my smart outfit? Hesitantly I followed her through the entrance. I was scared. What if the wretched fellow were to blab it out to all and sundry: "See that chap with Mistinguett? I had him thrown out of here for carrying bags without a licence." I was ashamed of having worked as a porter, then. I kept glancing round to see if the hall-porter was anywhere in sight, not knowing that these diplomats recognize people only when it is to their advantages.

That dinner with Mistinguett was my first experience of dining in style and I was feeling self-conscious. What with all those Englishmen in dinner jackets, I couldn't help staring. Amazing, how grandly these people dressed just to eat dinner. They were elegant enough, but why so somber? As for me, I was wearing blue trousers, a green jacket, and red shoes, and thought I was the last word. It was not until much later that I understood Mistinguett's comment when she saw my get-up: "Very good, Maurice, people will notice you." Certainly, had I been wearing a dinner jacket like everyone else, nobody would have remembered her anonymous escort. But such a bird of paradise dining with the great star is not so easily forgotten.

It was the first time I tasted caviare. I had heard of it, but I had no idea whether to expect a kind of sausage or a black pudding, a fish or a kind of omelette. I ate it without even knowing whether it was good—I had no standards by which to judge. It reminded me of the time my father ate oysters and everyone in the village had come to watch him. But here, nobody was watching me—the people at the next table were eating caviare themselves. I forget what we had for a main course, but I remember the crèpes Mistinguett, the coffee and the champagne. Mistinguett never drank anything else, but she ordered red wine for me, saying: "I know you don't like champagne." I thought she must be a mind reader, but of course it was only that she had known all kinds of men, including country bumpkins like myself.

Our meal was punctuated by a flow of advice: "Maurice, I've always patronized hotels that gave me a special price. Any hotel where I stayed could count on free publicity, and the bright ones saw it was in their interest not to charge me at all. But a person must have a secretary to attend to all these details. You'll soon be needing one yourself.

"You have a lot to learn, but I'm not worried about you. You'll soon pick it up.

"We're going to be interrupted all evening. I know a lot of people, and the ones I don't know want it to look as if they know me. They'll come to say hello, they'll be asking for autographs. Watch me carefully, I'll show you exactly how to handle them."

She was amazing, she calculated everything; her smiles, her gestures, the pitch of her voice when she wanted to attract attention, even the manner in which she introduced me:

WORLDLY: "Do let me introduce young Doctor Mességué. A magician, I've no more pain."

SUPERIOR: "Have you met the young Doctor?"

HAUGHTY: "What, you don't know Doctor Mességué?"

PARISIENNE: "Darling, an extraordinary boy . . ."

PATRONIZING: "Maurice, you'll see X or Y for me, won't you?" It was a dazzling performance.

I learned all sorts of things that evening—that waiters bring a little side-table to serve from, that hors d'oeuvres are wheeled round on a trolley, how to use a fish knife and a finger bowl, how to draw attention to someone, the niceties of social know-how . . .

"Do you realize that tomorrow the whole coast will know I was cured by a Dr. Mességué?"

"But they'll know I'm not a doctor."

"I never told them you were, I just called you Doctor. And there are all kinds of doctors about. Cheer up, you're going to be famous and popular and very, very rich. I'm never wrong, I have a nose for these things. I can always tell when someone's lucky."

She laid her hand with its load of rings on mine.

"Ask for the bill, I'll let you settle it."

I knew I didn't have enough money, but I went to the manager, Paul Andrès, to ask for the bill, which was staggering. My luck always seemed to run out at the Négresco."

"Look," I said, "I can only pay you half now. I'll bring you the rest before the end of the week."

"People don't come to a restaurant like this unless they can afford to," he replied.

"I didn't know a meal could cost so much. Besides, I thought Mistinguett had invited me."

My naïveté amused him. He knew his famous client as of old.

"That's a fine way to carry on, getting yourself invited out by ladies. Apart from that, what else do you do?"

I told him, and a few days later he and his wife became patients of mine. It was no longer I who had to pay.

I continued my frequent visits to Mistinguett, who always seemed glad to see me. She would talk about her life, about how she had started her career, and above all she would tell me how she felt she had been let down by Maurice Chevalier. She thought him very ungrateful, but I think he always remained the great love of her life.

"You see, he was just a Paris brat like me. We were nobody, either of us. We knew what it was to tighten our belts; we'd had plenty of rough times. You can't imagine what a handsome kid he was. The brute!"

She hated him like a woman in love.

Mistinguett was good-hearted, even kind, so long as you didn't ask her to spend any money. "You don't charge me, I know," she often said to me, "but look at what I've already earned for you." She was obsessed with money and harped on it constantly. "You must admit that having me for a patient"—it had been in the newspapers—"has put you in the limelight." In fact, contrary to what she thought, I was incapable of exploiting the publicity, of turning it to account. It's not enough to have certain talents; you must make it known that you have them if they're to be of use to anyone. But I was happy, it seemed to me that my success was stunning and my life marvellous. She wanted me to put some money aside, to buy some land—and that, with my attachment to the earth, was something I wanted too. Even before I had my first made-to-order suit, I had bought a few square yards at three or four francs a yard. Her favorite saying was: "You must be very careful with your money. You can never count on success like you can on money in the bank." She sent me several patients, among them a rising young star from the Casino de Paris, Colette Cereda, whom I luckily cured of hoarseness with one one foot-bath.

For me, Mistinguett stood for true beauty, and for a very long time she was my ideal of womanhood. She was tremendously desirable and tantalizing—and didn't she know it! She had plenty of common sense and she was kindhearted. Above all she was very much a woman—happily for her, for it was this that kept her young.

11

My First "Miracles"

W HEN I THINK BACK over the years 1947-49, I realize that they were the most extraordinary years of my life. Meeting Mistinguett had been a totally new experience for me. Through her I had encountered a whole new world, a world I'd never known existed. A multitude of new experiences followed, both personal and professional. I even had my first court summons!

People were no longer coming to me just for rheumatism, liver attacks, stomach disorders or poor circulation. I began to have scruples about treating many of my patients, and frequently asked myself: "What would my father do? Camille produced fewer and fewer answers—he had never been in a comparable situation, he had never had to face these difficulties, and yet I was convinced that "his" plants could do a great deal. I was to have miraculous proof of this.

One day I was called to Marseilles, to Dr. Bouchard's clinic in the Rue du Dr. Escarre, where an explorer named Varna lay dying. Before even looking at him, I naturally asked permission of the doctors in charge, which they granted with alacrity since, by the time I reached the clinic, the poor man had already been given Extreme Unction. When I saw him, so pale and dreadfully swollen, the crucifix upon his breast, my first reaction was to wonder what I was doing there. The doctors at his bedside brightened visibly—not of course at the prospect of the man's imminent death but at the sight of myself standing transfixed at the foot of his bed. They were as good as saying: So you're the miracle worker . . . Come on then, let's see you work one of your miracles now! One of them, however, was decent enough to draw me aside and tell me: "Listen, my boy, forget about this one. He'll be dead in an hour or two—he hasn't passed water for two days. It'll bring you nothing but trouble." I was fully aware of Varna's condition, for when I was first summoned to his bedside I had been told: "He has acute uremia. The blood urea has already reached a fatal level. His kidneys are completely blocked." And yet I had come. Was I mad? Who did I take myself for—Christ raising the dead?

To save time I had hired a car, and had brought with me a specially prepared compound of greater celandine, broom and the Watling-Street thistle which is given in the plant pharmacopoeia as the specific remedy for urea. With the coming of autumn, the heads of this "hundred-headed thistle," as it is also called, drop off and, carried by the wind, scatter their seeds far and wide. When the wind was rustling the dry brown leaves I often heard my father say: "The thistles will be off on their travels again. Who knows where they all come from or where they all go . . ." We use the root of the plant, which is recognized by the medical profession as being beneficial in the treatment of Bright's disease. In 1939 Dr. H. Leclere [1] made some highly interesting observations on its effectiveness in cases of congestion of the kidneys.

These were my only weapons against encroaching death. I stood there, looking at the dying man and wondering why I had come, fearful that heaven would punish my conceit. For the first time I was having to question my own conscience. I felt a lump in my throat at the thought that this man was about to die. I had never seen a dead man. I was filled with conflicting thoughts: "The man's dying!

[1] *Précis de Phytothérapie,* Paris. Masson.

Should I try to do something—or should I do nothing? If I walked out now it wouldn't harm my reputation; nobody could expect me to work miracles. If I treat him and then he dies, it could be damaging to me—I'd have made a fool of myself. The doctors know more about it than I do, and they say there's no hope for him, so who am I?" . . . I was still debating with myself when one of them asked: "Do you think you can get him to pass water?"

"Yes."

"If you do, it will be a miracle."

I might have answered: "For miracles, Catholics go to Lourdes, Mohammedans to Mecca, Buddhists to the Ganges, and Jews to the Wailing Wall. I'm only human, I'd better leave." Instead I heard myself saying: "I will take the responsibility."

I felt a sudden deep conviction that I could cure this man and at the same time I was thinking: "If you don't even try, you're a self-deceiving coward. If you don't have faith in your own treatment, you're a hypocrite." I took a pad of cotton wool, soaked it in my preparation and placed it over his kidneys. By now he had lost all feeling, his stomach was distended, his legs full of water. I waited. I think that was the longest half-hour I have ever spent. His breathing was barely perceptible—the sheet scarcely moved. If his heart stopped, all would be over. The others had gone, leaving me alone to watch over this stranger on the brink of death. After half an hour his urinal contained about half a tumblerful, and when I called the sister she exclaimed: "It's a miracle!" An hour later there was a tumblerful, four hours later, between seven and eight and one-half quarts.

This was twenty-three years ago, and Varna is still alive today. He was told all about it of course, as soon as he was able to take it in. It had been only a few years since he had to give up coming to court to testify on my behalf, as he is now an old man of eighty-five. As for myself, I have never again had to wrestle with my conscience in a case of that kind. I simply say to myself, the man is lost otherwise, so I must try. Even if there is only a chance in a million, I have to try. Plants can cure, but they cannot kill, and when all else has been tried, when orthodox practitioners give up, then it is my turn to do what I can.

I had not been back in Nice long when a Mr. Rameau, an engineer from Paris, came to see me. He had great difficulty in breathing and had to pause after every few words to recover his breath.

"Sir, I have come to you because in my view you are my last hope. I have already consulted all the top men in the medical profession, and I am neither temperamentally nor intellectually suited to trust in quackery of any kind. The doctors openly admit they can do nothing for me, so there is nowhere else left for me to turn. I chose you because you don't rely on some occult gift but on your plants, which I can accept as a possible scientific basis for your treatment."

The man was visibly exhausted by his condition, but nevertheless radiated tremendous energy.

"I've been a chronic asthmatic for over thirty years, ever since I was gassed at Ypres. My really bad attacks are so fierce that I've never been able to take up any employment, and when I'm not having an attack I'm in a state of suffocation. I have to sleep sitting bolt upright in a chair, and there are days when I can't even take a step up from the street to the sidewalk. It takes so much effort and courage and will-power just to go on living that I've more than once thought of putting an end to it."

This is only an abbreviated version of the man's troubles, for he talked to me for over an hour. It was clear that both his morale and his physical strength had been sapped almost beyond endurance.

There was no point in using my pendulum to examine him —in fact I never needed it to tell me what was wrong with a patient. For me, diagnosis is more an extension of my own intuition, a kind of sixth sense. All doctors have to rely on intuition, especially for diagnosis. Very often their experience, their scientific knowledge and their laboratory tests only serve to confirm the diagnosis made the moment the patient came through the surgery door. For Rameau my pendulum was to be of use principally in helping me establish my dosages, a method known as synthesization. My plant samples are kept in sealed glass phials. I move the pendulum over them while remaining in contact with the patient, and, according to the amplitude of its oscillations, I decide on the proportion I should use. The plants are not a random assortment but a selection I have previously made and am now merely modifying. I had not been using this method for very long, and certainly never before in connection with so serious a case as this asthmatic.

With asthma, as with all manifestations of allergy, one is to a large extent groping in the dark. Often, success can be attained only through a process of trial and error. In this case, anti-spasmodics being of prime importance, I selected medicinal lavender, meadow sage, greater celandine, and the corn poppy, rather than the opium poppy, because its narcotic effects are milder and more easily tolerated. I also included wild thyme, which acts powerfully on the respiratory apparatus and more particularly on wet asthma (bronchial asthma), in conjunction with parsley, which is an excellent expectorant. Finally I greatly increased the proportion of ground-ivy, a humble, pretty little plant which has nothing in common with any climbing ivy. I use only its stems. In the seventeenth century many doctors attributed to it anti-consumptive properties, which it is far from possessing, but in 1876, Dr. F. J. Cazin, one of our best modern experimenters in the use of wild plants for medicinal purposes, declared that he had cured cases of chronic pulmonary disease solely with the aid of ground-ivy. My father used it in the treatment of anything to do with the respiratory tract, and it invariably gave good results.

After half an hour I gave my patient the prescription for his foot-baths. He read it and looked at me:

"Will this—do you honestly think this will make any improvement? Will it give me some relief?" He paused and then added humbly, "That's all I ask."

"There is every reason to hope so."

"I believe you are an honest man. You're not just saying so?"

"No, I mean it."

To tell the truth, I was really sticking my neck out, and was a little frightened at assuming such a responsibility. A few weeks later, Rameau began to feel a real and distinct improvement. We hardly dared to believe it, either of us, for in asthma, remissions are frequent, particularly when there is a change of treatment. But in his case the improvement held, and three months after his first visit he came to see me again.

"Now I really dare believe I'm cured, and I've come to thank you. I promise you won't find me ungrateful."

I might be a newcomer to the trade, but I was already familiar with that kind of talk, it never led to anything. It was only much later that I heard that my friend Rameau—for my friend he became—had written a letter to a Paris weekly with a wide circulation:

Gassed during the 1914-18 war, I had suffered ever since from asthma, so badly that in 1920 I had to give up work. Recently my condition worsened to such an extent that the doctors advised me to try anything if I thought it might help. Maurice Mességué treated me with plants, and cured me. My condition has so improved that I think I can go back to work.

I'm a civil servant, and therefore not the kind of man to take kindly to anything unorthodox. But my conscience tells me I must let people know how I was cured. Do we, you and I, have the right to let people suffer if there is truly a possibility that they might be cured as I was?

The printer's ink was barely dry when the effects of this letter became apparent; it was even partly responsible for my first summons. Rameau's visit had certainly proved significant. Only a few more months of peace were still left to me, if you can call peaceful the hectic life I was leading: commuting between Nice and Menton, gathering my herbs, giving consultations. However, I had found the time to send for my mother. As soon as I saw that I could count on ten clients a day, I had written to her: "Take off your apron, you're not going to work for other people any more. Come and join me here." Ten clients was the target I had set myself. My mother had toiled all her life, and I wanted her to be able to take things easy at last. She was so happy when she came, but she was shy too, and at first the sight of all those people waiting for me in Menton or at 5 Avenue Durante alarmed her.

"Are you quite sure you know what you're doing? What if these people cause trouble for you?"

My own place wasn't big enough for her to live with me, so I had found a room for her, and she was happy. "I'm living like a lady," she would say, "with all this sunshine and all these flowers. It hardly seems right!" Life had so knocked her about that even to this day she is anxious, almost fearful, so much so that I still keep her in ignorance of my social life. This part of my life frightens her a little, for she herself has remained the humble peasant woman from Gavarret, the wife of Camille.

Several weeks after Rameau's last visit I met the young woman who was to prove the turning point in my life: Anne-Marie Moraldo. When she entered my consulting-room in Menton my first thought was, "she can't have come to me for treatment!" She was a pretty young woman, well-rounded, glowing, fresh, healthy, as full of life as a Mediterranean flower. Her hair was dark and her eyes had that velvety luster you find only in girls from this part of the world, eyes that are full of promise yet never brazen. But then I saw that she had a withered arm bent back upon her breast like the wing of a wounded fledgling, and this caused her to hold her head a little to one side.

"I've come to you because my father, who works for the post office, heard some people saying you were a kind of healer, so you see . . ."

She pointed to her arm. Yes, I saw, and it was enough to make you weep, she was so lovely.

"You'll do something for me, won't you? You won't leave me like this? I'm nineteen, you see . . ."

"Have you seen any doctors?"

"Have I seen any doctors! I've even been to Lyons to see them. And they've left me as I am. At first they said, 'It'll get better when she grows up.' Now that I have, they say, 'You must be patient.' Patient! My patience is exhausted. Tell me, do you suppose I could ever find a man to marry me with this?"

There were tears in her eyes, and she avoided pronouncing the word arm. I didn't have the courage to say, "I can't do anything for you. My plants are as strong and as simple and as beautiful as you are yourself, but they can't work miracles."

"What . . . how long is it since your accident?"

"It wasn't an accident. I was born like this."

Start by treating what? The nerves? Certainly—and then?

"You look as if you're thinking the same as all the others. You aren't going to give up, are you? You'll try?"

Yes, she was right, I had to try everything.

"Does your arm hurt?"

"Yes, whenever it's going to rain."

So it wasn't completely without feeling.

"But I don't feel anything except the pain in my bones. They've scratched me and stuck pins into me and I don't feel a thing."

I was thinking fast. Rheumatic pains . . . we'll need diuretics to eliminate any poisons: wild thyme, stinging nettle, great burdock and parsley. Anti-spasmodics, relaxants to calm the nerves: common camomile. Mild sedatives—very important to help her sleep and relax: hawthorn and linden-blossom. Now for the atrophy, let's see, it's really a kind of rickets, so we'll try field-horsetail. (Animals that can barely stand on their feet, even when close to a state of collapse, can be successfully treated with field-horsetail combined with cabbage and watercress, which are also stimulants and known to be effective in cases of anemia.) And I'd better add some root of cross-leaved gentian and some onion.

I had chosen the plants with almost clinical precision but, I wondered, was that enough? After all, nature had made this young woman the way she was, and I was opposing nature with nature. Would I succeed? I really had no idea. I made out a prescription for poultices and foot- and hand-baths.

"When should I come again?"

"In three months, when you've completed the treatment" —I had prescribed a particularly long course of treatment —"or sooner if you notice even the slightest improvement."

"Oh, thank you, I'll let you know at once, if you're sure I won't be a nuisance?"

"Not at all! Don't hesitate to come and see me." I wasn't running much of a risk saying that, I thought.

"You've given me fresh hope."

I was afraid that was all I had given her. She left me with a new doubt: "What if after all I'm only a purveyor of hope?" But no, I had cured, I had even saved . . . Poor kid, the good fairies certainly hadn't been present when she was born, but perhaps the good fairy of the plants would help her now.

Some weeks later, at about three in the afternoon, I opened my door to admit the next patient. A tall, thin young man was just walking out.

"Where are you going?"

"I'm just leaving."

"You're in a great hurry."

"It's just that I don't need to see you any more."

"Even so, would you mind stepping inside?"

Insolence is one thing guaranteed to make my good Gascon blood boil.

"Are you suddenly better, then?"

"No, there's nothing wrong with me. I've learned all I need to know."

"What about?"

"Your activities."

"But who are you?"

"Henri Mari, a journalist."

When the Paris weekly received Rameau's letter, they had decided to follow it up and had sent their local correspondent to see me and question me.

"Then why are you leaving?"

"Because I heard through the door the advice you gave your last patient: linden-blossom tea with orange blossom! An old wives' remedy, as everyone knows! You've got your nerve, taking money from people for a bit of advice that isn't even a proper recipe!"

"I took no money from her, you're wrong about that. There was nothing I could do for her."

"That hardly surprises me. I thought as much. I've seen all I need to see, I'm leaving."

"You've seen nothing."

I might well have lost my temper and thrown him out, but for some reason I took a liking to this angry young man, all boiling over with integrity and righteous indignation.

"Sit here next to me, as if you were my assistant, and perhaps you'll 'see' something," I told him, and I called in my next patient.

When you know someone is critically observing your every move, it isn't easy to talk to people and listen to them and try to understand them, for this demands total absorption, a degree of concentration that doesn't come readily to me at the best of times. When you're studying someone with the pendulum, the presence of a hostile stranger makes your task no easier. I began to wonder what idotic pride had induced me to persuade this boy with the cynical smile to sit beside me. To make matters worse, as far as I could tell I didn't even have the advantage of being any older than he was.

"Well, I've got these pains in my back, about where the kidneys are, you know what I mean, and I've taken all kinds of stuff, but nothing does any good. And then I get kind of a burning sensation in the pit of my stomach. And my right arm's almost too stiff to move."

The poor fellow was getting ridiculous, and I was thinking, if he mentions his feet I'll burst out laughing. The very fact that I was harboring such thoughts—I, who have such total respect for my patients—shows how much on edge I was. I wanted only to get rid of the man, so I gave him an embrocation for rheumatism and also a poppy sedative and mint for his stomach, and showed him out. Henri Mari was smiling, and clearly wouldn't have staked a penny on my chances now.

"You know he's no more sick than I am! And if he's cured he'll come and tell me? What's that supposed to prove?"

I didn't have time to answer, and whatever thought was in my mind was instantly forgotten: Anne-Marie Moraldo had just entered.

"Yes?"

"I've come to say hello."

She held out her hand. Not at the usual level but chest high. Nevertheless her arm was free.

"Look ... I can ..."

She leaned down and picked a sheet of paper off my table.

"Your hand ... you can use it?"

"Yes, I am so happy!" she cried, and began sobbing like a child. "It's so marvellous, I can hardly believe it. It was this morning ... I ran and ran ..."

I felt like weeping myself, and my eyes were stinging as I blew my nose hard and stammered: "I . . . I'm so very pleased. Tell me . . ." I had forgotten the journalist and his insulting scepticism. He could go or stay as he pleased, I couldn't have cared less.

"Is it all right for me to talk in front of this gentleman?"

"Perfectly all right."

Far from threatening to leave, he was listening intently.

"I didn't feel anything the first month. My father kept saying, 'He's just another quack, that fellow.' (I'd heard that before!) The second month I began to feel a kind of tickling sensation, as if a sort of strength was returning to my arm and my hand. I'd never felt anything like it before. And then little by little it began. I could move one finger, then another. Every day I did exercises, but I didn't say anything to anyone. I wanted to be sure before I came to see you. And here I am."

"Do you mean to say that you couldn't previously move your arm and your hand? That Mességué treated you and now you can?"

"That's exactly what I'm saying."

"And are you sure?"

"Of course, I'm sure. Don't you believe me? Hold out your hand."

He did so and she pinched him several times, with some malice.

"Can you feel that?"

"Distinctly."

"Well then, so can I. And it's thanks to Mr. Mességué. He's given me the finest present I've ever had in my whole life. It's my birthday today, I'm twenty."

The next day Henri Mari—who has become a very dear friend—started his investigations. Mr. and Mrs. Moraldo told him: "That man is a saint. What he did was a miracle. He saved our daughter." This was moving but not very conclusive. So he went to see the doctors who had examined the young girl. One said: "Medical science cannot at its present stage hold out any hope regarding the reanimation or cure of an atrophied upper limb. Various treatments, particularly radiotherapy, can be tried without danger, under medical control." Another: "Nothing can be done. It is beyond the power of any doctor to correct congenital deformities."

But the proof was there: Anne-Marie was using her arm and her hand. Henri Mari pursued his investigation to the end. I might conceivably have paid the Moraldos to attribute to me a cure due to some other intervention, so he made enquiries in their district, only to be told that they had in no way altered their way of life. The police reported most favorably on the morals of both daughter and parents, and everyone he questioned—friends, teachers, employers—told the same story. Finally he consulted a specialist who provided him with the "reasonable" explanation he was looking for:

"It could be that the use of external agents, physical or chemical factors acting in conjunction with certain psychic elements, might have effectively modified the tissues and motility of the organ."

Then Henri Mari submitted his report to his newspaper—twenty-five typewritten pages—which concluded:

"I no more believe in healers now than I did before. Maurice Mességué is certainly no sage who has discovered some new therapy. But one thing must be admitted: he has helped people for whom medicine can do nothing.

"It may be that his work defies both law and logic, but the fact remains that he does heal."

Yes, I was a healer, and now I no longer doubted it.

12

"My" President

I THINK IT WAS July 26, 1948. On every street corner were
posters advertising the Congress of the Radical Socialist
Party at the Municipal Casino in Nice. There was something
pleasingly French and festive about this Congress, and the
list of "star attractions" on the poster was impressive. Heading the bill was the retiring President, Edouard Herriot,
Mayor of Lyon. A real gala program. Of all the names there
was just one that fascinated me, Edouard Herriot, and I had
decided to go and hear him speak.

For a long time now my views about politicians had been
changing. Far from being uninterested, as I was once, I
now felt myself very much drawn to them, realizing that
these were the men who made history. The greatest of them
all, in my opinion, was Herriot, the champion of the people.
He was in the same class as Jaurès—all of whose speeches
I had read—and in the same tradition, with his ringing de-
livery and speeches full of ideas and information.

The thought struck me that, since he was actually there,
why should I be content just to go and listen to him? Why
not ask to see him? Pleased with my decision, I went up to
a little group of men at the Casino door who were check-
ing admittance to the Congress.

"Good morning, gentlemen, I've come for the Congress."

"Where are you from?"

"I live here, but I come from the Gers."

"Where's your rosette? And your admittance card?"

"I haven't got one."

They stared at me. I was thin as a lathe and garbed in a rather worn maroon polo-neck sweater and a pair of electric-blue trousers. I thought it was quite a smart outfit, but it couldn't have been the ideal uniform for a member of Congress, since they refused me admittance.

It must have been two or three days later when my doorbell rang at 5 Avenue Durante. I opened the door and saw before me the rather saturnine figure of a man dressed entirely in black except for his very white collar, which was so stiff that it made him hold his head rigid.

"Mr. Mességué?"

"Yes," I said, thinking that the man must have come to serve a summons on me. For quite some time people had been tipping me off "in confidence" that my "activities" were unpopular with certain doctors.

"Let me introduce myself: Friol, Head of President Herriot's Cabinet."

"Please come in," I said, too stunned to think any further.

Standing stiffly in the middle of my room, on a mat that was threadbare—as I now noticed for the first time—Mr. Friol, after throwing a glance of polite surprise round my "surgery," said: "President Herriot would like to see you urgently. Can we arrange an appointment?"

President Herriot! I was paralyzed. Meanwhile, Mr. Friol, with all the warmth of a high-class funeral director, went on to say: "As President Herriot had to leave immediately after the end of the Congress and his re-election as leader of the party, it will be better for you to examine him in Paris."

In spite of his diplomatic impassivity, there was nothing very flattering in his expression as he looked round my humble abode. Sitting there, on chairs that didn't match, we eyed one another with a great show of politeness: "Do you

mind if I look at my diary? I have a great many appointments, especially in Menton."

"I have no doubt. But the President can't get away, and
you will be able to examine him more comfortably in his
home. I will send you your ticket for tonight's train, and a
car will be there to meet you at the Gare de Lyon. And . . ."
—he had lowered his eyes and was looking at my shabby
canvas pumps—"I've been instructed to tell you that you're
not to worry about expenses."

I flushed at this, but it was all my own fault. I was earning enough money to dress properly and buy decent shoes,
only I never thought about it. Certainly, if clothes make the
man, then I looked a poor specimen.

As soon as Friol had shut the door behind him, I tried
to collect my chaotic thoughts. To treat President Herriot,
me! What ailment could it be? Certainly he must need to
lose weight. They said he was a big eater. As well to check
his liver perhaps. It could be that he had arthritis, rheumatism . . . What if he had something else? I was not a chemist,
I couldn't pick a remedy off a shelf and take it with me. I
had a few basic preparations, but I modified them for each
case. Sometimes I had to allow twenty-four or forty-eight
hours before giving a patient his preparation, since this was
the time it took to macerate semi-fresh plants when I
thought them necessary. It was equally clear to me that I
couldn't go to some unknown shop in Paris and buy desic-
cated herbs that would have lost two-thirds of their virtue.
I had to have my own plants, I had no confidence in any
others, and so I crammed my suitcase with plants and bottles.

With my suitcase full of plants and my personal effects in
a bag, I arrived at the station a full two hours before the
train was due to leave. Peasants from the Gers always believe in being early—and despite all the lessons Mistinguett
had taught me, I was a peasant again that day all right! I
traveled first class, which for me was a novelty. It was hard

to believe that I was actually going to see, even treat, Herriot himself. How could he have heard of me? It could not have been through the popular weekly that had written me up—had someone recommended me? I was quite on edge with suspense and got very little sleep; three hours at most. At Laroche-Migennes they were selling coffee in paper cups on the platform, but although I was longing for some I didn't dare get off the train in case it should leave without me.

When I emerged from the Gare de Lyon and took one look at Paris, I knew at once that it wasn't my kind of place. It was too big. Driving through the streets in the rather grand limousine that had met me, I could see that it was a beautiful city, a city with a soul no doubt, but a city that in no way appealed to me. We drove along the *quais,* crossed the Seine, which I found very grey indeed, and drew up at the Hotel de Lassay,[1] a very pretty little town house. I could take nothing in. I felt dirty and crumpled, though I had done what I could in the way of a wash and brush-up on the train, and the chauffeur had instructions to take me straight to the President. At the door of his room I wondered nervously what to do with my suitcase —I could hardly take the thing in with me.

"Put it down there," I was told.

The speaker was a dark-haired, wiry little woman of about sixty, whom I at once realized must be Césarine, Herriot's housekeeper, thanks to the newspapers a celebrity in her own right. She gave the impression that, with her on the job, the President was well-guarded indeed! She looked me over and missed nothing.

"Come along then, follow me."

You could tell she'd said "come along" just like that to plenty of people before me. And so I was shown into the President's room, which nearly took my breath away. It was a huge room full of old furniture heaped with newspapers

[1] Residence of the Presidents of the National Assembly.

and books and garments. The drawers in the chests were open, and on a bed, like an island of flesh in an ocean of bedclothes, sat the President.

I was totally unprepared for the sight. I was expecting to meet the Mayor of Lyon, President of the National Assembly, the man who the day after the Liberation had refused the presidency of the Republic, the biographer of Beethoven and Madame Récamier, the friend of Alfred Cortot the pianist, the man of letters, the scholar, the most cultured of conversationalists. But what I saw was this huge man on his bed, in a crumpled nightshirt that barely reached his thighs—his gargantuan thighs!

He was looking at me. His eyes were sparkling with mischief in the shadow of his black eyebrows, his mouth firm and kind beneath his short moustache, his broad bull-like forehead deeply furrowed below his short, wiry hair. He was somehow larger than life and yet reassuring. Around him were gathered several grimly important-looking gentlemen.

I waited uncertainly.

"Let me introduce the healer Camaret has sent me." Hearing the name, I was at once less nervous; it was one thing less to worry about. I later learned that at some time during the Congress in Nice, Herriot had complained to Dr. Camaret of his rheumatism, and the doctor had told him: "My wife got rid of hers, I sent her for treatment."

"Was she treated by one of your colleagues?"

"No, by a healer."

"A quack!"

"No, since he made her better."

"And what's his name, your magician?"

"Mességué."

But that morning in the President's room I knew none of these details.

"Come closer, Mességué. What a young creature he is! Say good morning to these gentlemen. They've been taking care of my rheumatism for years! Have a good look at them—they're the worst bunch I ever knew, worse than a bunch of Communists!"

In their cold, ironical glances I could read what they were thinking: A quack, the President's gone as far as that, has he? He's getting senile. They left the room with dignity, and I found myself alone with Edouard Herriot. I was thinking fast; I couldn't afford to make a mistake. But it wasn't difficult to diagnose the trouble.

"Mr. President—do you weigh yourself often?"

"Never, my boy. I hate upsetting myself!"

While I respectfully passed the pendulum over him, I questioned him. I was more at my ease now; doing my job always gave me confidence.

"What do you have for breakfast?"

"A nice big milky coffee and a few croissants."

I thought it better not to inquire how many.

"*Apéritifs?*"

"Only a few."

"Lunch?"

"You know, I was born in Troyes on the borders of Champagne, and I'm Lyonnais by adoption, so I am obliged to make a few 'sacrifices.' Could you imagine a Mayor of Lyon who didn't appreciate *quenelles de brochet,* the *poularde demi-deuil* of la mère Filloux, hot sausage, *foie gras en brioche,* Burgundy and suchlike good things? I'd lose my job."

"How many hours a day do you work?"

"My boy, I never count anything."

"Women, either?"

"I no more count beauty than I count time or money."

"And you have pains here and here and here."

I pressed firmly on the painful spots. He bore pain with courage, but in his eyes I could see the old familiar anguish of the suffering.

"What will you be able to do for me?"

"First we'll ease the pain, and in a few weeks you'll be walking without a stick. You'll be able to lead a normal life.

You must take two foot-baths a day, morning and evening. Tomorrow I'll bring you a bottle of my preparation, which you'll pour into the water."

"And will your baths stop the pain?"

"My father always obtained good results."

For a Gascon, that was a real Norman answer!

"Why can't you give me your wonder potion right now?"

"Mr. President, I have to make it up for you."

"Don't you give the same thing to everyone with rheumatism?"

"No. While I was examining you with the pendulum I was also testing, with the help of these little tubes, which plants would be good for you."

"And where are you going to buy them?"

When he heard that I was trailing my suitcase full of herbs around with me, he gave such a mighty roar of laughter that he shook all over.

"I shall have to believe in you, you're so obviously sincere."

"You're sincere." For hours I couldn't get the words out of my head. I had opened my suitcase and was trying to work out my dosages, but I was making no headway. I had lied to the President. Foot-baths wouldn't be enough; he would have to go on a diet and I hadn't dared tell him so. I'd been afraid of losing my patient. I could see it all quite clearly now—I wasn't treating a patient, I was treating President Edouard Herriot. Meaning someone who would help me to "arrive," someone who would be good publicity for me. And I felt ashamed. It hadn't taken long for "success" to turn my head.

I was perhaps going to alleviate my patient's pain, and it was possible that this would bring me a certain reputation. But from that moment on I knew I had to set all vanity aside. There's no more merit in treating a famous man than any other. I still had to make up my preparation. In Herriot's case, relieving the actual pain came second. First I devoted all my care and attention to the diuretics—field horsetail, sour cherry stalk, beard of corn—and to the plants that are both diuretic and anti-rheumatic: great burdock, onion, meadow-sweet, creeping couch-grass roots.

It is sometimes very difficult to determine which will be the most effective diuretic for a particular patient. Certain plants have very complex properties that can either heighten their effect or produce the very opposite; the onion is one such plant. It has a long list of properties—diuretic, stimulant, anti-scorbutic, expectorant, antiseptic, resolvent, anti-rheumatic—and is therefore an excellent remedy for constipation and flatulence, chilblains, sores and whitlows. In short, it would seem to be a universal panacea that can be used quite safely. But this is not so. Dr. Cazin advised against it for anyone of an excitable or worrying disposition, for persons subject to hemorrhages or suffering from shingles. There are people with liver disorders who cannot tolerate it. Relatively recent research has shown that while its high sulphur content makes it effective against rheumatism, it could become harmful in liver cases where there is an allergy to sulphur.

One of my doubts that evening was whether or not to include onion. Although a powerful enough diuretic for one to have seen it clear the kidneys of patients with uremia, and an excellent treatment for rheumatic pains, it could lose its effectiveness altogether and even become dangerous if the President's liver couldn't take it. The pendulum had reacted favorably, but as I didn't consider it a magical instrument or believe in its absolute infallibility, I decided against including onion.

At the thought of facing the President next morning and standing up to him over the question of a diet, I once again spent an almost sleepless night in my fine room with its soft carpeting and heavy drapes. The next day, I found Césarine more friendly.

"What are you going to do to Mr. Herriot?" she asked.

"I'm going to put him on a diet."

"My poor man, you might as well pick up your suitcase and go. He'll never keep to a diet!"

Too bad, I thought, but my mind was made up. I found the President sunk in his pillows and evidently in pain, and I looked on him now simply as a patient.

"Quick, let's have your bottle." He held it in his stubby, powerful-looking hand. "What have you put in it that hasn't been in the stuff I've already been given?"

"I don't know. A great many remedies are based on plants. But I can promise you one thing—you won't find the slightest trace of any chemicals. My herbs have grown free in their chosen soil, where nature intended them to grow. They were happy plants, and that's important. When you're happy you're at your best."

"It makes sense, what you say, and it's a nice idea. So then, you're going to cure me?"

"No, Mr. President, but I'll make you better."

"Does it interest you to know that my rheumatism is neither progressive nor chronic?"

"Not much. I'm not a doctor. It isn't the kind of rheumatism you have that I'm going to treat. It's you, my President."

"What do you mean?"

"I mean that I treat the patient before the illness. You have rheumatism because you eat too many good things and too much of them. You are carrying too much weight and so your body has to be constantly making an enormous effort. You lead a sedentary life and your system is poisoned. You'll get no better if you go on eating all those dangerous foods you told me about. I like *foie gras* myself—they make the best *foie gras* in the world where I come from—but I don't eat it every day of the week. You must eliminate one meal, preferably the evening meal, and replace it with leek broth and unseasoned boiled greens. You should drink only water."

"You can't do this to me! It's murder—and you're asking me to agree to it!"

Césarine was right, I thought, this would never work. My career in the world of politicians was going to end here. Too bad! I must have been looking fairly dismayed, for Herriot gently patted my hand.

"Don't look so miserable. I've decided to do as you say. It'll make Césarine happy at all events, she's been at me long enough with her 'Go on a diet!' "

After two months of this strict treatment, Herriot was walking without a stick and had lost twenty-two pounds (10 kilos). I hadn't abandoned any of my patients in order to treat the President, and so I had to ply to and fro between Lyon, Paris and Nice. It was tiring and also depressing, for I could see at a glance every time he put on weight! My triumph was short-lived, for two months later we were back where we'd started: the President had put on twenty-two pounds.

"Mr. President, are you keeping to your diet?"

"My little Mességué, how could you doubt it?" he said truculently, "you can ask Césarine."

I had no need to ask her, for Césarine came to me of her own accord.

"My poor friend, there's no point in my making him good vegetable broth and watching him make faces as he eats it. He's deceiving us both. I'm a light sleeper and the other night I heard a sound in the kitchen. I had my suspicions so I crept down quietly, and there he was, our President, sitting at the corner of the table eating a tin of *foie gras* with bread and a nice bottle of Burgundy."

Césarine wasn't the only one to inform me of Herriot's excesses. Mr. Friol had confided to me in a more diplomatic style: "Dear boy, do you know why the President prefers to travel to Lyon by car rather than by train? So that he can pay a gastronomic call on Dumaine at the Cote d'Or."

I knew well enough what that meant. I had seen Herriot,

at the banquet of the Radical-Socialist Congress in Toulouse, eat his way through *foie gras,* a magnificent cassoulet—of which he had three helpings—Roquefort, plum pie, washed down with Bergerac, Bordeaux, coffee and brandy, and finish off with a nice fat cigar. Besides, I happened to know Friol was telling the truth. One Saturday I was driving through Saulieu when I spotted the presidential car in the car-park of the Relais de la Cote d'Or. I went in to say hello to the President, and saw him sitting in front of a steaming plate of coq au vin, sniffing the delicious aroma with half-closed eyes. As soon as he saw me, with incredible dexterity he whipped off his plate of coq au vin and set it on the neighboring table, which was occupied by an English couple gravely eating egg salad, and he grabbed one of their plates in exchange. Of course, I pretended not to have noticed.

"Egg salad, young Mességué, there's nothing like it for the health!"

"You're quite right, my President."

It was six o'clock in the evening and time to leave, when Herriot sent for the maître d' hôtel and said: "If there's any left, I'd like just a little more of that cassoulet!"

He had the same hearty appetite in everything. One day when I was with him on one of those last visits to Saulieu, he vanished just as we were about to leave. We looked everywhere for him. We went up to his room, but he wasn't taking a nap. Alarmed at the memory of the gargantuan dinner he had eaten, we looked in the toilets, but he wasn't there. We ran out in the street calling "Mr. President! Mr. President!" Friol was white as a sheet and wondering whether we shouldn't send for the police: "He might have taken sick, he might be lying somewhere. How can we find him?"

It was the chauffeur who found him, in a basement room in the company of a lovely, strapping wench. At seventy years of age! What's more he was laughing at the good trick he'd played on us.

"Mességué, you're not going to forbid that too!"

You couldn't forbid him anything, in fact. I still wonder how I had managed to get him on a diet in the first place. Really, he was a force of nature. Everything about him was huge: his laughter, his voice, his body, his intelligence, his cultured mind, his benevolence. He wasn't on the same scale as the rest of us. It wasn't easy for me to struggle with him. My reproaches made him laugh, and the only thing he took seriously was my plants.

"At least *they* do you good without asking anything in exchange! Your only mistake with me, Mességué, was to think you could get me to put them in my stomach too!"

At times there was something deeply touching about this man who refused to grow old, who refused to lose his gusto and with it all the good things of life. When he used to say to me: "Don't say I can't, let me be happy. At my age it's too late, sacrifices don't pay dividends," I couldn't help giving in to him, nor growing fond of him. He was a person of great warmth and kindness. I used to call him my "number one tout" since, thanks to him, there was a moment when I had treated seventy-five deputies, which prompted him to remark: "My dear Mességué, don't forget me when you have your majority in the Chamber!"

In appearance he put you in mind of an ageing bull, but in his friendships he showed all the delicacy and modesty of a young priest. When we were chatting together he would break off to think aloud: "I must remember to tell one of my friends, who's suffering from———, that you might be able to help him," and he never forgot. He always expressed his views mildly, starting with "I'm one of those who think that . . ." and never "What I say is . . ." or "My opinion is . . ."

I often went to see him in the morning while he was still in bed—which was permanently hollowed to the shape of his heavy body—and he would talk to me about all kinds of things: about men—and about women. He was very fond of women: "Can you imagine a world without women?

Think how sad and ugly it would be. Love's the most beautiful thing in the world!"

My own ignorance of politics he found particularly amusing. "You might have done well in politics," he said, "because you don't understand the first thing about it, which is an excellent position to be in, perhaps the best!" Once he talked to me about France, and he spoke strangely, more as if he were talking about a much-loved woman or a mother. These rambling conversations of ours were far removed from the vigorous presidential speeches that roused parliament to life.

He spoke to me about our "top men" as he would have spoken of his parents, trying to understand them and excuse their mistakes. He considered Daladier as a brother who has strayed along a different path, and Blum as a cousin-figure, highly estimable but distant. De Gaulle? "An interesting fellow. He's cramped by the political framework we have today. But he's a very good Frenchman, and I believe he's an honest man." His only criticism of de Gaulle was for the trial of Pétain. "I think that had I been in the General's place I'd have chosen a different policy. I didn't much care for Pétain; he was rather a limited old man but not a traitor. To bring the nation together I think de Gaulle would have done better to make his peace with him."

Our longest discussions, however, were about religion.

"Tell me something, Mességué. Lourdes isn't far from your part of the country, and people do say that miracles happen there. You dabble a bit in these things, what do you make of it?"

"Mr. President, I don't mind admitting to you that I love the Holy Virgin. I even prefer her to the Good Lord himself. She's a woman, a mother, she's more indulgent. We're all of us her sons, in a way."

This made Herriot laugh indulgently, and I was encouraged to continue:

"I often go to Lourdes, although not during the height of the season, when that collective hysteria is being shamelessly exploited by people who make a living out of other people's suffering, with those devotional objects flaunted for sale wherever you look, those temple merchants holding the floor. I'm revolted by people who prosper on suffering and religion. Yes, I'm with you there, Mr. President. That's the kind of thing that puts me off the religion of the priests. But people are cured at Lourdes, no doubt of it. Miracles? I don't know whether the cures at Lourdes are religious miracles, because there are plenty of equally miraculous cures taking place elsewhere. I was recently brought a little girl of four who couldn't speak, and now she uses over a hundred words. Mr. President, do you believe that it was only my herbs that cured her?"

"What do you think?"

"I don't know. But I've spent a lot of time carefully studying the big dossiers of the miracles of Lourdes, and they taught me a great deal. What struck me as most significant is that an apparently incurable case, with the patient maybe even on the brink of death, can be cured other than by orthodox medicine. It isn't always easy to be an outsider, to work without the protection of proper diplomas. You can't help having doubts, and so it reassured me to think that all those people miraculously cured at Lourdes had consulted good doctors, but they hadn't had the luck to meet a doctor who had faith. I have a great belief in the power of faith, whatever its form or origin or cause. And I am equally sure that it takes two: both patient and healer must possess it. Our greatest doctors are men who themselves believe in medicine, even if they know its limitations, and they, too, work miracles."

"But where does God fit into all this?"

"I think it was Ambroise Paré who said something like 'I only dress their wounds, it's God who does the healing.' "

As time passed, each time I saw my President, I found him more and more preoccupied with the idea of God.

"My dear Maurice, I'm one of those people who don't believe in God, but I have nothing against others believing.

Every man should do what he wants. What I dislike is the unwarranted interference of the Head of a Church in the politics of a country. Isn't God above all this?"

I felt that Herriot still had the same lively mind and sharp intelligence, but that in his sick body his soul was troubled. What man could not give him he was seeking elsewhere, in a higher place, blindly. He kept coming up against the idea of God, and he couldn't leave it alone. I had the impression that it was now tremendously important to him.

"You see, Mességué, I think I'm like good old La Fontaine. I've never had much time for the church, but you'll see, I'll die religious yet!"

On the threshold of death he abandoned little by little his old atheism. When a sick man can no longer believe in medicine, what else can he believe in? This was doubtless why on March 6, 1957, at the Saint-Genis-Laval clinic, the President received Cardinal Gerlier, primate of the Gauls.

I am a peasant, as firmly attached to the things of this earth as anyone, but even so, I say that it's harder to die a materialist than a believer.

13

My First Court Case

IF I WERE TO CHOOSE a family crest, I think my motto would be "I love." I love life, mankind, sunshine, plants, flowers, women—and I love my work. It has given me my greatest joys and also my worst torments, which only goes to prove how much I love it.

These thoughts were in my mind that February morning in 1949 as I was walking on the mountainside near Sospel. The sun had not long risen, and in two hours I would have to go down to my Menton consulting-rooms and forget the mountain and the sky and the fragrance that surrounded me, intense and heady, so typically Mediterranean. I would have time to think only of my patients, who, with growing frequency, gave me cause to question my own conscience. My life had changed in the last eighteen months. I had had to solve a great many problems, and often enough I had had to make arrangements on the spur of the moment. My visits to the President took time, and whenever I was away for two or three days I felt guilty about all the people who were waiting to see me.

Gathering my plants was another problem. I had so many patients that I could no longer be sure of finding the time to replace my stocks of herbs myself. I had tried getting help, but the people hereabouts are spoiled by living in the town; they lack the knowledge and devotion of the peasants of the Gers.

I made a lightning trip to Gavarret, to look for elderly people who would know how to handle plants and who would also have that knowledge of nature that comes only with a lifetime of experience. I started setting up a system of gathering and drying plants which, although I have made some improvements, has never been substantially altered.

It wasn't a simple matter to arrange, and I had to make several visits. My plants cannot all be picked in the same way or at the same time, for there is a favorable month and a favorable time of day for each one. They lose their goodness if they are picked in the wrong season or at an unfavorable moment, or if they are growing in poor soil or are improperly dried or kept for too long. The first rule is never to pick plants along main roads, where they are poisoned by exhaust fumes, nor pick plants that grow close to cornfields or orchards or vineyards, where they can absorb the harmful spray of chemical fertilizers or insecticides. Plants must be picked as far away as possible from land under cultivation.

I have them picked where they grow wild, where the process of natural selection results in stronger, richer plants nourished by their chosen soil. For the gathering of each plant there are rules that must be respected, rules that vary according to whether one is picking the flower, the leaves, the stem or the root. Plants are particularly rich in sap in the morning and roots in the evening. "It's because of the plant's circulation," my father used to say, "its blood goes round just like our own."

Flowers, stems and leaves should be picked as soon as the dew has evaporated. Flowers such as hawthorn should be gathered while they are still like young maidens, before they have bloomed into maturity. This is very important: the flowers of the common broom, one of our best diuretics, can cause gastric disturbances if they have been picked when they were turning into pods.

Many plants are best gathered in the summer solstice, around midsummer day, as our forefathers knew. The weather should be neither too damp nor too dry. Roots must first have all soil removed, then be quickly washed and brushed before drying. The actual drying of the plants is of prime importance, for on this depends the extent to which plants retain their effectiveness. It is all a question of touch. Plants should be neither too dry nor too fresh and never completely dehydrated. The initial drying should be done in the shade, never in the sun, in a well-ventilated but never a draughty spot, away from insects, and the plants should be spread out on a sheet, and turned at frequent intervals. After this they can be "finished," an operation for which a sieve is ideal, since it allows air to circulate freely. The most usual method, however, is to hang the plants in little bundles, heads down, inside the house.

For a long time I have had a house in Gavarret full of herbs, its beams and rafters covered with hanging bundles. My plants are the sole inhabitants of the house, and they have their own watchman who opens the windows for them in fine weather, shuts them when it rains, and locks them up every evening. He's been looking after them for twenty-five years.

Lastly, the dry herbs should be stored out of the light, for light drains the color and some of the goodness out of them. Certainly, plants will go paler or darker when they are dried, but providing they have retained their color I can guarantee that they are still potent.

I also had to evolve a method of packing and sending the plants. At the beginning they were sometimes useless by the time I received them, either moldy because they'd been packed too fresh, or nothing but a heap of dust because they'd been packed too dry. Such mishaps were not only disappointing, they were disastrous, for how could I tell people, "I've run out of plants, come back next week —or the week after? I couldn't. How are you supposed to explain to people twisted by pain that you'll ease their pain —but later?

My various problems had barely sorted themselves out

when a new cloud loomed on the horizon. Many people were coming to me, my success was arousing jealousy in certain quarters, and I was warned by people whose motives were perhaps doubtful that I was being "watched." I disliked the expression—felons and wrongdoers were "watched"— and I couldn't for the life of me see what harm I was doing by treating sick people, often free of charge.

Dr. Camaret, who was the president of the Menton Medical Association, had once warned me: "Watch your step, you're becoming too successful. People are talking. My colleagues aren't all like me. There are twenty-six doctors in Menton, and you're getting more patients than any of them." Dr. Echernier, whom I had seen again and even treated for rheumatism, had also put me on my guard:"Maurice, you aren't liked. I warned you, it's a jungle here on the coast. People think that because there's plenty of sunshine there'll also be plenty of gold, and they come pouring in from all sides. By the time they discover that life here is just as hard, if not harder, than anywhere else, it's too late. So then the claws are out; it's the struggle for survival. Doctors are no better and no more easy-going than other men, I'd hate to have to testify for you in a court of law."

"A court of law?" I remember answering. "You make the world out to be worse than it is. I'm not doing anybody any harm and that's what matters."

Gradually, all these "kindly" warnings were beginning to get on my nerves. I couldn't see what anyone could have against me. I'd put myself right with the State, being duly licensed to practice radiesthesia, and with the Pharmaceutical Association, since I never charged for my bottles of preparations. It would never have entered my mind to sell God's plants. I was at peace with the doctors and with my own conscience, since I never treated a patient without taking all kinds of precautions. I was only twenty-nine, but I knew my limitations as well then as I do now. I never took it upon myself to diagnose a condition, but started by ask-

ing the patient for his doctor's diagnosis. I am very intui-
tive, and I admit that this sixth sense, so to speak, often
gives me very useful guidance in my work, but I never
rely on it completely. I have always been mindful of the
fact that, though they might not necessarily know more
about patients, doctors know more about illnesses. I have
never presumed to declare "this man is suffering from so-
and-so," nor have I ever disputed a doctor's diagnosis and
substituted my own. It may be that, by my choice of plants
and the dosages, I modify or amplify the original diagnosis. This is because I am treating the cause prior to the
effect, but the patient does not know this.

I never accepted cases that orthodox medicine or surgery
are better equipped to handle effectively. I did not take it
upon myself to treat typhoid or any infectious disease, nor
did I aspire to cure tuberculosis or cancer. I never put a
patient in danger, and I was so afraid of making a mistake
or overlooking something important that whenever a patient
said, "I haven't been for any tests, it's not worth it," I
would send him directly to one of the three top doctors in
Nice who were willing to work with me, for all the necessary tests and X-rays. To my mind, the first thing in medicine
isn't to cure but to avoid doing any harm! That I pro-
ceeded with such caution was not for fear of some spying
policeman but because my own conscience would have
been uneasy had I failed in the least degree to act correctly.

All these thoughts were milling through my mind as I
made my way downhill to Menton, but I wasn't at all worried. Despite the "kindly warnings" given me by my friends
and others, I wasn't prepared for what came next. I didn't
believe it could happen. Even today, when I think back to
that February day in 1949, I remember it as one of the
hardest days of my life.

That day, in the middle of a consultation, I was handed
a yellow envelope containing a summons to appear in court
on a charge of practicing medicine illegally. Infringement of

the statute on which this summons was based rendered one liable to a fine of one dollar to ten dollars and imprisonment for two months to two years.

I was overwhelmed. I went on seeing patients all day, looking at each as if at a dear friend I was forced to desert in an emergency. Some of them were new patients, and as I examined them I was thinking "Luckily his treatment will be short, he won't need me for long," or else "how will he manage, his treatment will take months?" For, emotionally involved as I tended to be in everything I did, I expected I would be made to stop my work; I felt shattered. I remember a woman saying to me that day: "Without you, Mr. Mességué, what would become of poor folk like me, when the doctors won't have us any more?" Her words so echoed my own thoughts that I think I almost hustled her out, which was unlike me.

I was all the more wounded because that wretched bit of paper specified "at the request of Dr. Camaret, President of the Menton Medical Association." In the bus on my way back to Nice I went through the whole gamut of emotions —rage, disgust, an urge to fight, and finally resignation. After all, I could always get a job somewhere as a schoolmaster again. But I was choking with rage at my helplessness in the face of what I considered an injustice.

That evening I was seeing Suzanne Jaffret, who later became my wife. I was already very much in love with her. She had come to me a few months before to ask for treatment, and I had fallen in love with her the moment I saw her. I didn't dare to tell her. I had always made it a rule to look upon my female clients only as patients, and so each time she came I would say to myself, "I'll ask her to have dinner with me when she's cured. But her treatment dragged on and on, and I began to worry and question the value of my plants. I couldn't know that she was fibbing so that she could continue to see me, thinking that once she was better she'd no longer have any pretext! That evening we had arranged to meet and I told her all about the summons. I think I talked at length, at great length, which isn't like me. While I have the southerner's easy manner, I also have his profound reserve. I seem to keep nothing back, but I never speak about things that are really close to my heart.

"Have you rung Camaret?" Suzanne asked.

"But he's the one who's attacking me."

"You know perfectly well that it can't be him. You should go and see him, and also have a lawyer to defend you. Ask your patients to back you up—you can't just give up."

She was quite right, of course. The next day I saw "good Dr. Camaret."

"I tried to warn you, but I could not reach you. I had no choice. Out of twenty-five doctors, twenty-one asked me to take action, but it doesn't mean I'm not on your side, and I shall be of more assistance to you yet."

"I'd certainly have been surprised if it had been the other four; I'm treating their wives."

Brave words and I believed in them. But I was beginning to realize quite clearly that as far as the law was concerned I would always be an illegal practitioner, a kind of secret operator. I would never officially be granted the right to heal, I would be given formal notice to give up my activities indefinitely, by people of the same ilk as the headmaster in Bergerac. My life would become a chronic self-contradiction. On the one hand, men like Edouard Herriot and a number of doctors would recognize my abilities and accord me the right to heal, while on the other hand there would always be people ready to harry me and keep me from doing my work.

As for the actual proceedings! P., the division superintendent of the judicial police in Nice, had sent me "patients" who were in reality police informers ready to testify that I was practicing medicine illegally—a pointless undertaking, since I made no secret of my practice. When Superintendent P. took me in for questioning, I answered every one of his innumerable questions, but there was one, had he asked it, that I would have refused to answer on the grounds of professional secrecy, namely, "Does my mother come to you for treatment?" As she had been coming to me quite a while before P. entered my life, I have never known whether it was he who advised her to come or whether she came on her own.

It's not in my character to give up without a fight, and so I had prepared to do battle, but when I crossed the threshold of the law courts in Nice on April 28, 1949, I was feeling profoundly discouraged, and I'd decided to give up after the hearing. Mr. Pasquini, who was conducting my defense, said to me: "I promise you that this case will go against them in the end. You'll obviously be found guilty, the judge will be obliged to enforce the law, but I have no doubt that you'll come out of it the real winner!" But all I could think of was that I was being taken before a court of law, and that if my father had been alive, it would have made him ill. I was bringing shame on the Mességués.

Mr. Pasquini had called 228 witnesses, but the bench decided to hear only 50 of them. They were all eager to go up and say their piece, describing their sufferings in simple language. It brought a lump to my throat to hear them—and I certainly wasn't the only person in that courtroom to be so deeply affected. No one could help being moved by the little old lady of seventy who had dressed in her best clothes to come. She scuttled over to the witness box like a little mouse, and only she and I knew that those rapid, pattering footsteps were a miracle.

"Would you like to be seated to give your evidence?" the judge inquired.

"Oh, no, I can stand up all right now." Speaking slowly, carefully choosing and weighing her words, she went on:

"Well, for two years I hadn't been able to walk. Not a step. I had to keep to my bed, and I was all alone. My children are out in the Colonies, and I didn't want to go to them. A helpless old woman like me is a burden to young people, Your Honor. Eventually all my savings were used up. I didn't want to ask the children for anything, it would only have worried them. They gave me injections, massage, electricity, rays. They weren't bad doctors, they didn't see any harm in selling me some hope, and of course they didn't know that in order to pay them I was living on bread and two cups of coffee a day. The eleventh doctor I saw told me: 'It's no use, you must be brave . . .' I thought he was talking about my death, and I told him, 'Don't worry, I'm not afraid to die.' What he said then was worse for me. 'You'll never walk again.'

"That gentleman there," pointing to me, "came to see me. He gave me the first foot-bath himself, and he's never let me pay him anything. He treated me, and you can see for yourself how well I can walk. I've got the proof here, all the certificates," and she rummaged awkwardly in her black handbag, with her shaking old hands. "Your Honor, for people like us who've been given up by the doctors, that man there is like the Good Lord Himself. Don't hurt him. Without him there'd be nothing left for us but to die."

A Swiss, Mr. Peyrot, had travelled all the way to Nice to say:

"Your Honor, I had consulted more than twelve French and Swiss medical practitioners, all capable men, but none of them was able to relieve my attacks of asthma. I was suffocating day and night, and Maurice Mességué cured me in five days."

When my little Anne-Marie M.'s turn came, and she held out the hand that had been paralyzed, fluttering it in the sunlight and moving it away from her body, the judge involuntarily exclaimed: "But it's a real miracle!"

In the courtroom women could be heard sniffing and blowing their noses.

Next to be heard was the mother of little R., from Chateauneuf-de-Grave: "My little boy, Your Honor, was like a zombie. He could walk and run about like other boys, but it was as if he were separated from life—he didn't seem to hear and he couldn't speak. Not a word. I was the only one who could understand him. When he grunted I knew whether he was happy or sad. I'd learned to read his eyes, they'd grown so big they seemed to devour his little face. Perhaps they were taking the place of his two missing senses. So I had nothing to lose when I heard people talking about the 'Miracle Doctor.' I took the boy to see him, and when he started talking about soaking his hands and feet I thought he was kidding. I was mad! But I was too unhappy even to swear at him and tell him he was a quack. And then my little boy held out his arms to him, he trusted him. I thought, children often sense things we can't, and I decided to try the baths. We haven't been doing it for long, Your Honor, but my boy has been talking for a month now, and yesterday"—Mrs. R. burst into sobs—"I'm sorry, it's just that I'm so happy, yesterday he called me 'Mama' for the first time."

These witnesses actually caused quite a stir in the courtroom, but even more astonishing, both to me and to the bench, was the evidence given by Doctors Camaret, Echernier and Leroy, who had dissociated themselves from the action brought by their colleagues. Doctors defending a healer—such a thing was unheard of.

"Doctor, we are listening."

Dr. Camaret made his statement: "Maurice Mességué does heal. The first client I sent him was my own wife. He cured her rheumatism, from which she had been suffering for twenty years. None of us had been able to bring about any improvement. I subsequently sent him certain patients considered incurable and he has either brought about some improvement or cured them completely. These results are undeniable."

Dr. Leroy declared: "Not only are his plant treatments effective but, being applied only externally, they are in no way dangerous to the patients."

Dr. Echernier had sent his written testimony: "I certify that as a result of following the course of foot-baths prescribed by Mr. Mességué, I was almost miraculously cured of a rheumatic condition which had troubled me for several years and had failed to respond to all other treatments."

After the twenty-eighth witness had given evidence, the party bringing the action announced that it was not contesting the effectiveness of the treatments, so no further witnesses were heard. To Mr. Pasquini this meant that we had carried the day, but I was not so sure. When I saw Mr. Montel, prosecuting attorney representing the Medical Association of the Alpes Maritimes, rise to his feet, I had a feeling that the hearing was about to take a very different turn.

"As a lawyer," he began, "I am here to argue against him, but as a man I am quite ready to take his foot-baths to cure my insomnia! We are not contesting Mességué's cures. We intend to show only one thing, that he is illegally practicing medicine. He heals, but he has no diploma entitling him to do so. He must therefore be found guilty."

And I was, to the tune of ten dollars damages awarded to the Medical Council, and thirty dollars damages to the Menton Medical Association.

At the foot of the steps outside the law courts, in that old quarter of the town where I had so often wandered penniless, quite a crowd was waiting for me.

"Well, Mességué," Mr. Pasquini said, "now you're famous."

I couldn't have cared less. I wasn't interested in fame that depends on scandal.

"Come along, Mességué, don't be so gloomy. For these people, you're a legal blunder—they acquitted you long ago!"

He could well have been right, but my decision was made: I was giving up. Meanwhile the crowd had advanced up the steps, people were holding out their hands to me, touching me, clutching at me. Out of the general clamor my ears picked up odd words and snatches of phrase: "We're with you." "Bravo." "My son is ill." "I'm desperate." "Remember me." "I'll come tomorrow." "Give me an appointment." Obstinately I shook my head: "No, no, I can't." For me it was all over. The words, "He has no right to heal because he is not a qualified doctor," were ringing in my ears. No, for me it was no triumph, it was a defeat. I had been under the illusion that all would turn out well, but now I knew that I would always be up against the law, that I would never be granted the right to heal. I would give up.

I didn't sleep much that night. Morning found me with stubble on my chin, an aching head, and a bitter taste in my mouth. It was barely daylight when the *concierge* tapped on my door:

"Mr. Mességué, they're here, they're waiting to see you."

"Who?"

"Patients, more than a hundred of them."

"I'm not seeing anyone."

"But you must! There are old people, women, children . . ."

Losing my composure I yelled, "I don't have the right—understand? I don't have the right!"

There was a woman with the *concierge*, and behind them I could tell there were others. She was a very ordinary woman, wearing overalls, and she looked straight at me: "Sir, it's not possible, you can't do that to us—you . . ."

She was right, I couldn't do it.

"All right then, come in."

14

Doctor's Pupil

I OFTEN SAY THAT MINE is the finest job in the world, much as a cabinet-maker might say of his craft. A man has to be sure that his job is the best and finest for him, or he will have no confidence, he'll always feel he's in the wrong shoes. There is nothing sadder or more depressing than a man whose heart isn't in his work. I make a point of asking everyone who comes to consult me: "Do you like your job?" It's so important for the morale; a patient who is happy in his work is always much easier to cure.

Were I to be prevented from healing, I couldn't be happy. I believe I was put on this earth to heal, and if I didn't believe this, if I had only been doing it for the money, I would have given up long ago.

The day before the hearing I felt very successful with my thirty patients a day. The day after, I had more than a hundred, and each day I was getting more than five hundred requests for appointments. This could hardly have been the result looked for by the Medical Council! When evening came a great many patients had to go away without my having seen them. There were children and old men and women, and people with walking-sticks and crutches, and they begged me: "Sir, I've come two hundred, three hundred miles and I can hardly stand up!" "The child is tired." "Don't tell me to come back." By ten o'clock that night I was exhausted. I'd had nothing to eat, and still there were just as many people at my door.

On those evenings I felt afraid. I would go out on to my little balcony to have a breath of air and look at the night, feeling that it was all too much for me. How could I possibly measure up to their confidence, their faith? I am only a man, I can be wrong. Will the empiric knowledge of the Mességué's always be enough?

I think it was on the eighth day that my wife—Suzanne and I had got married—came to me: "Maurice, this can't go on any longer."

Unhappy as I was, I gave vent to an outburst of rage—the usual rage of frustration over an insoluble problem; directed as usual at the innocent—and I shouted: "I will not let them down!"

"You don't have to, but you must get organized. You must find a larger apartment, hire a secretary, start thinking about looking for an associate, someone who can look after the basic prescriptions and the bottling of the preparations."

She was right; to continue as I had been was madness.

"You don't have the time to cope with all that. All your thoughts and your energies should be for your patients. If you like, I'll take care of all the practical details."

In a few days she had found us a six-room apartment at Cimiez in the Majestic, a palatial establishment originally built for the English but now past its heyday and converted into apartments. I liked its situation, in a quiet district overlooking the town, a kind of Neuilly in Nice which suited me perfectly. My wife played a very important part in my career, for I was—and still am—a disorganized person, and she was exceptionally good at organizing. She engaged secretaries, as I could no longer keep up with filing patients' cards and answering letters and making appointments. The first time I was able to reply: "See my secretary," it gave me the feeling of being a free man at last. Best of all, she spared me the job of asking for fees. I hated having to hold out my hand to take money. I had found it hard to do even when I was working as a porter. It didn't help to tell myself that this was different; I never could get used to it. I also tried to avoid being thanked by patients I treated free of charge; I found it very embarrassing. Whenever I sense that they've saved up their pennies and made needless economies to come and see me, I don't enter any figure on their card, so when at the end they ask my secretary for their bill, she tells them: "Nothing."

One afternoon a ravishing little woman, Mrs. B., came briskly into my consulting-room. She was slim and blonde, and I noticed that she was wearing elbow-length gloves. Hm, I remember thinking to myself, that must be the new fashion. She sat in such a way that I saw only her profile, and she spoke without turning her head. Her voice sounded weary: "Sir, I know you ask patients for a note from a doctor or a specialist, so here's a letter from Professor R. that will tell you all about my case."

A fine phrase but not quite accurate. The letter informed me that the doctors were giving up Mrs. B. because hers was an obstinate case of "vitiligo with achromia and hyperchromia." I hadn't the faintest idea what the words meant, but I could hardly say so.

"Tell me how you first noticed the trouble."

"When I was looking at myself in the mirror. See for yourself—look at my face, my hands."

She had white blotches on her skin, like bleached spots, surrounded by dark areas.

"So far I've had them only on one side of my face, but now they're starting on the other side too. It isn't just personal vanity. I'm a saleslady in a fashion house, and I can't possibly go on with a job that brings me in contact with clients who set such store by appearances."

Two months later she was cured, and Professor R. confirmed the disappearance of the bleached patches.

The same day a man of about sixty came into my office, leaning heavily on his walking-stick. Walking obviously cost him great pain. He, too, handed me a letter from a specialist, along with a bundle of X-rays.

"They don't convey anything to me, all these X-rays and notes full of medical words, but you'll know what it's all about; you'll be able to tell me whether it's serious and whether you can cure me."

The specialist's letter and the notes with the X-rays were highly technical:

Lumbar myelogram
Reveals no hernia.
Small protrusion in L4-L5.
Marked shrinkage of cecal pouch due to swelling of posterior wall.
—in: L4-L5
    L3-L4

Cephalic rachidian fluid
Sugar:	0 g 50
Albumen:	1 g
Chlorides:	7 g 20
B.W.:	negative
Red corpuscles:	204 per mm3
White corpuscles (Leukocytes):	1 per mm3
Bacteriology:	negative
Culture:	negative.

What lay behind all those words? Perhaps tuberculosis of the bones, an illness I refused to treat. Ought I to send him back to his doctors? Fortunately a few moments' conversation made it clear that he was suffering from lumbago and sciatica in his right leg, so I felt sure my foot-baths would bring him relief.

This was a new problem to me, because so far I had worked only with doctors who knew me and spoke a language I could understand. They would express the results of their tests in simple everyday terms, concluding with: "I think you might be able to do something for this patient," sometimes even going so far as to say: "I think it helpful to warn you . . ." But now I was getting patients from farther and farther afield—Marseilles, Valence, Lyon, Paris, Lille, Strasbourg—and even from abroad: Belgium, Switzerland, Holland. Every day I was coming up against what my father used to call "learned" words. I was being handed reports I couldn't understand, medical phrases that might just as well have been written upside down for all they conveyed to me. If I tried to look knowing in front of the patient, it wasn't from vanity but for fear of alarming him, of making him think, The fellow knows no more than I do. I have never made a secret of the fact that in many cases the effectiveness of my treatment has stemmed from the patient's confidence in me. Now my ignorance of medicine and medical terminology was proving a great disadvantage, and I decided to remedy the situation: I had to enlist the aid of a doctor who could teach me all I needed to know.

I went to see Dr. Echernier and confided my problem to him:

"I can't go and sit on the students' benches in a medical school, so what should I do?"

"You must have had an idea in mind when you decided to come and see me?"

"Yes. You're very learned, you're head of a teaching hospital. Would you be willing to give me some lessons?"

He looked at me with his cool, piercing blue eyes:

"Why not? You're an honest lad or you wouldn't be here now. I know you're already earning plenty of money, but you evidently don't think that's all that matters. You've had enough success to give you quite a fine opinion of yourself. But you came. I like that. When do you want to start?"

"At once."

"You haven't changed a bit! Right, then, let's get started. I'm going to begin with the most elementary but also the most fundamental thing of all: how a man is made, how the machine functions. Then we'll have a look at the things that can go wrong and what causes them to go wrong."

I worked with him four or five hours a day, although how I managed to find the time I don't know. Whenever Suzanne said: "You can go now, that's the last patient," I didn't argue. Even if I saw people who looked as if they might be waiting, I didn't stop. She was able to say no to them, but I couldn't.

I marvelled at osteology and myology. He taught me the meaning of polyarthritis, neuritis, arthrosis, radicular neuralgia. Until now I had been like my father. I'd known only the word "pain." Studying with Dr. Echernier I began to acquire more than a rudimentary knowledge of medicine. The lessons taught me a great deal about the progression and complications of diseases and the symptoms of certain conditions, but above all they taught me the need for great caution, and a healthy fear of medicine. I began to realize just how dangerous medicine can be, and when I hear of babies being treated for eczema with shots of cortisone, or year-old infants being given barbiturates, I have no hesitation in calling it criminal folly. The study of medicine taught me, above all, the need for humility in medical work and the need to recognize that our surest knowledge is that we know nothing. So many times I have known patients to go to three or four doctors, all capable and honest men, only to wind up with as many different diagnoses as doctors. This is why I say that medicine is an art, not an exact science.

My life now was a whirlwind. I was getting letters from Paris saying: "You're so far from here, the fare's very expensive." "I can't come to see you because I can't leave my work." "Set up a practice here." And so I did, at 5, Place de la Parte de Champerret, in an apartment obtained for me by Mr. Rameau, who had been one of my first important cures. Next came Lyon—the Lyonnais reckoned I owed it to them, since I was treating their mayor! I liked this rather frenzied activity.

In retrospect I can see that the life I was leading then was harmful. Excessive activity becomes a kind of drug. I grew addicted to it, and now, for all the odd-week retreats I steal at La Trappe, I have lost the art of relaxing. If I am not up and doing something, I feel guilty. To think that I am the son of Camille, who knew how to take time to observe and teach me, in order that I might become what I am.

My appointment books were filled for three months in advance, famous names side by side with unknowns. What saved me from becoming a "fashionable" healer was that in my consulting-room I made no distinction between the patient who arrived on foot and the patient who stepped out of a Rolls. Disease is a great equalizer.

One sunny autumn afternoon the Baroness Hauser came to see me at Champerret Place. Sixtyish, elegant, well-cared for, she might have been definable as a typical woman of her class, except that she was wearing a most untypical necklace of pearls so enormous that I thought: "If they're real, this must be one of the wealthiest women in Europe." I wasn't far wrong: her husband was a banker. In their establishment in the Avenue Gabriel in Paris they had no fewer than twenty-seven servants, and their hunting preserve in Spain covered some forty-three miles, as I learned subsequently. I found the Baroness rather on the defensive, politely ironic: "Your reputation, Sir, has led me to think that you might perhaps be able to help me."

"Madam, did your doctor give his permission for you to come and see me, or did he actually advise you to come?"

"Not that it makes much difference, but I'd say he gave his permission."

"It makes a great deal of difference from my point of view, Madam. If he merely gave his permission, then you have come here thinking, After all, why not? But if he advised you to come, then you believe I can cure you."

She smiled: "Yes, I see."

"What is your trouble?"

"This will explain better than I can." She handed me the results of an X-ray examination. She had a fully developed arthrosis in her right shoulder, with secondary arthrosis in the cervical vertebrae.

The pain in my shoulder is so bad that often I can't sleep. I entertain and go out a great deal, but I daren't wear a low-cut evening dress unless I want to pay for it for hours afterwards—and they can seem very long hours." Then developing what was by now a classic theme to me, she added: "I've tried everything . . . I've been to specialists . . ."

I prescribed much the same treatment of poultices and foot-baths that I had recommended to Admiral Darlan, and they proved equally effective. For her I had also included in my preparation hawthorn, which is excellent for general circulatory disorders, particularly in women, and sage, which is a wonderful anti-spasmodic.

"How often will I have to come?"

"Only once, Madam, to thank me when you're better."

I knew quite well that the Baroness had come to me because I was in fashion, and she imagined that as I must be aware of her great wealth (which wasn't so; her name had conveyed nothing to me), I would spin out her treatment.

One morning Dr. Claoué's secretary telephoned and asked to speak to me: "Mr. Claoué would very much like to meet you. He leaves it to you to suggest the day and the time."

Claoué was the pride of the Gers, a highly skilled and much respected surgeon who specialized in cosmetic surgery, and I have always felt drawn to anyone who is, in one way or another, an artisan of beauty. When you mention cosmetic surgery, people tend to think of women having a face-lift, and often forget about facial injuries such as occur in accidents or war, or unfortunates whose disfigurement is such that it can cause grave psychological damage. If I were asked who were the men I should most like to meet, cosmetic surgeons would have been high on my list. So I could hardly wait to meet Claoué, and when I first saw him I was a bit surprised: a handsome, attractive face, warm, sparkling, black eyes, white hair, an intelligent head set on a body that was barely man-sized. He was short, just over five feet tall. His hands were remarkable, unforgettably fine and strong, and his fingers were the fingers of an artist, which he knew, and he would laughingly say, "I've got fingers like a fairy, that's why I've taken up sewing!"

"Ah, there you are. So you're from Gers too? Tell me about yourself."

From the start his tone was friendly and informal, but I had such respect for his knowledge and his authority that I felt intimidated. I told him something about my background and more especially about my latest ordeal in court.

"Don't be on the defensive, I know you're an honest man," he told me. It appears that without my knowing it he had been sending patients to me. "And you always acted courteously and correctly towards them. You've never taken advantage of the situation and made them pay unnecessary visits." He had pushed the experiment a stage further by sending me a patient suffering from disseminated sclerosis, a disease for which medicine has no cure. Remissions can be long, but the outcome is always fatal, and it is one of the conditions I have never attempted to treat. I remembered the patient clearly, for she had been a very beautiful young woman and her tragic case had moved me deeply.

"So it was you who sent her. I was very grieved when she died."

"So was I. I know that you honestly and openly refused to treat her, but I also know that you often went to see her and lent her your moral support right to the end. To me you're a true healer worthy of the name. I have important plans for you which we'll discuss presently."

That evening as I returned home I was walking on air. A great doctor, Dr. Claoué, had said to me: "You're a true healer worthy of the name." To me, this was the success I had been hoping for all these years.

15

Lord and Lady X

I HAD PASSED my driving test and bought myself a Citroen, which I was very fond of, and which in no time had become indispensable to me. Together we sped along the highways at mad speeds, for I had discovered the pleasure of driving fast, too fast—although always with a clear conscience, always with the good excuse that I was hastening to see a patient.

One night, when I returned from Lyon, my wife said:

"You have to call Mr. R. in Marseilles immediately. He left his number."

"The kind of illnesses I treat can always wait for a day."

"Ring him anyway to put his mind at rest."

Mr. R. must have been waiting for my call because he replied at once:

"At last, it's you, Mr. Mességué. My little daughter is terribly sick. The doctors have agreed that I should send for you. I beg you, don't lose a minute . . ."

The man spoke so brokenly that it was all I could do to understand him.

"What is the trouble?"

"They don't know, Sir."

"But . . ."

"Do you have children of your own, Mr. Mességué?"

"Not yet."

"Try to understand. My wife can't take another night. She can't stand it any more . . . and my daughter . . ."

"All right, I'm on my way."

So I set off again. It was a mild night, and I drove with the car window open to keep myself awake. Driving through the state forests in the Maures, the car was filled with the scents of Provence, and what with this heady fragrance of plants and flowers and my own tired and overactive mind, my heated imagination began to conjure up all kinds of thoughts and images. I felt "powerful and alone," I saw myself alternately saving the child or else unable to prevent her from drifting into the sleep of death, with the scent of incense.

I don't know how long it took me to reach Marseilles, but I certainly made record time. The father was waiting for me in the hall of their beautiful house, and I saw at once that they were clearly very rich people, among the richest in Marseilles, as it turned out.

"Our family doctor is with her now. Come this way."

"Just a moment, Sir. Tell me what's the matter with her."

"We don't know. Fifteen days ago she came back from winter sports complaining of a sore throat. Our doctor said it was a touch of tonsilitis, but for days her temperature hasn't dropped below 102°F. We've tried everything, we've tested for everything, but still her temperature doesn't drop."

"And there's nothing else wrong with her?"

"Nothing."

My enthusiasm was waning.

"Take me to her."

The doctor in charge, Doctor M., was more like a friend. He'd even sent patients to me, so he welcomed my presence. The young patient, a pretty little dark-haired girl of seventen, looked a little weary, but not seriously sick. Her mother, on the other hand, was in a pitiful state. Doctor M. drew me aside:

"We can't make head or tail of it. She's been examined

by three of my colleagues and by a consultant. It's a curious fever, it doesn't rise or fall, but this in itself is no indication. Her pulse is not the usual febrile pulse, nor is it, however, symptomatic of typhoid. There seems to be no immediate danger, but the girl won't be able to withstand such a high fever for very long. In cases like this the temperature can shoot up alarmingly. Listen, your plants can't do anything against this fever, you can refuse to treat her."

He left me alone with the girl. When I held my pendulum over her, it oscillated with a vigor that denoted the best of health.

"You're not a doctor?"

"No. But, tell me, do you feel anything?"

"Yes, I feel hungry! They've put me on a diet and I lie here dreaming of grilled perch and garlic mayonnaise and chicken . . . ," and her eyes sparkled in her pale, round little face. I felt her hand. It was barely warm. This child had no temperature of 102°, she was in perfect health.

"Well?"

"You aren't ill at all."

I thought she was going to leap out of bed.

"You're marvelous!"

This was hardly the opinion of Doctor M. His expression changed entirely. He became hard and aggressive and really almost nasty.

"I thought you were a good honest chap, but there's nothing good or honest about what you're doing. You're sneering at her parents and you take us for a bunch of idiots. We might make a wrong diagnosis, but we can hardly make a wrong reading of a thermometer."

We stared at one another, the same thought suddenly entering our minds: what if there was something wrong with the thermometer itself?

"I've never once encountered such a thing in all my twenty-five years' practice," he said. "But I suppose anything is possible . . ."

I had no more suspected that this might be the explana-

tion than he had, but being unencumbered by science I
had at least been sure of one thing, that the girl was not
ill. Ten minutes later the girl's father was on his way to
an all-night chemist for a new thermometer. In fact he
bought two, to be on the safe side, and by four in the
morning I was back on the road, leaving our patient hun-
grily devouring a chicken leg. Her temperature chart showed
only 98.4°.

The few souls who might have seen me driving through
Marseilles that night must have thought I'd taken leave of
my senses, for I was convulsed with laughter as I drove
along. Still, I was aware that such a mistake—so easy to
make in medicine, with its rigid faith in its rules and
instruments—could in some circumstances be anything but
a laughing matter. Doctors, for the most part, could be
counted on to take all kinds of precautions and perform
all kinds of tests and analyses and to consult with each
other. But how about the others, the quacks? The fake
healers? I could see very clearly just how they would have
taken advantage of such a situation, and I was well aware
that there is nothing to distinguish a true healer from a
fake. Cleansing the Augean stables was certainly going to
mean a struggle, and would need the support of the medical profession. Why not a man like Doctor Claoué? So my
thoughts were humming in my head, in time with the regular humming of the engine. Already on the horizon the
night was growing paler, the air was cool, and the scents of
the countryside were numbed, for like me they need the
sun's warmth to bring them to life. I felt myself sinking into
a kind of well full of cotton wool which took on the form
of a serpent stretched out ahead of me like a road . . .

My dream ended against a wall not far from Fréjus.
Stunned by the impact, I went on seeing slow-motion images, I was burying myself in darkness and silence. The
sound of the engine had stopped. I wasn't in any pain, I
just wanted to sleep. Then I heard shouting and saw flames,
I tried to open the car door but a searing pain paralyzed

my shoulder. The dream was a nightmare now. Men's voices were shouting: "Get him out!" "He'll be burnt alive!" "Watch out for the gas tank!" Hands dragged me roughly out of the car. Gradually I regained consciousness. I was in pain and my beautiful new car was in flames . . . but I was saved. I owed my life to some soldiers from Fréjus who had been out drilling on the road: without them I would have been burnt to death.

A dislocated shoulder and two broken ribs were all I had to show for a thermometer that hadn't worked . . . but after all, I told myself, it was one of the risks that went with the job. I'd be running other risks before I was through. I hadn't forgotten the idea that had been uppermost in my mind that night—the notion of publicly defending my profession—and I'd been to see Doctor Claoué, who had been encouraging in his own way and had promised to help:

"There's too much talk about you. You have so many patients and chalk up so many successful cures that it's like an accusing finger pointing you out to the Medical Council. Whether you keep silent or whether you speak out, either way they aren't going to leave you alone, so you might as well say publicly whatever you have to say. Begin by giving lectures to explain your ideas and defend your work, but don't start attacking others, not yet. First separate the wheat from the chaff. I'll be right next to you whenever I think my presence might be useful."

"But I don't know how to talk."

"Get away with you! You're from the south, a Gascon; where we come from you start talking in your mother's womb!"

I accepted the idea, but I imposed strict rules on myself. I never take the initiative; I wait to be invited to lecture; nor do I give treatments in the locality where I am lecturing. There must be no suspicion that I may be acting as a salesman for my own professional services.

However, I did give my first lecture in Nice, in the Bréa

Hall. I suffered acute stage fright. I had never felt so small in my life. Sick at my own audacity, I could only think: "You're going to look an absolute fool standing by your table with your glass of water." My worry proved ground-less; I knew my subject inside out. When I started speaking someone shouted, "Louder!," so then I really let myself go. When it was over I felt quite pleased, not so much because of the applause but because I had managed to say all those things that had been choking me ever since my prosecution, particularly this:

"Those of us who are called healers want only to be able to heal in peace. This the Medical Council will not allow, and if a doctor is known to be co-operating with us, then he is prosecuted along with ourselves.

"We ask permission to treat the patients given up by orthodox practitioners while accepting, even asking, their supervision of our treatment. Even if a healer has only one chance in a hundred of curing a patient, should this be denied him? Why should he be punished for it? Nobody has the right to refuse a patient his last chance. Let me ask one question: when doctors refuse a patient this last chance, where they themselves have failed, are they really acting in accordance with the Hippocratic oath?"

It was a success. Within a few months I had spoken in more than twenty towns, from Antibes to Paris, from Rouen to Bordeaux, from Toulouse to Lyon. The lecture I gave in Algiers, which was held in a big cinema, turned out to be a real gamble. I had been warned that there would be doctors present in the hall, but this didn't worry me, for more and more doctors were attending my lectures by then, asking questions which were only rarely spiteful. That day, however, as I began my talk I felt a kind of anxiety. It wasn't so much fear as the feeling that something was going to happen. The hall was so crowded that the people were even overflowing on to the pavement. It was a hot country, a land of passion. The people listened, they let me speak, but they commented to each other on whatever I was saying, which created waves of sound eddying out into the street and echoing back to me. At the end, at question time, a man stood up and said:

"Mr. Mességué, I am a doctor. You haven't spared us much, but what I say is that you know a bricklayer by his wall. In your case, you know the healer by his patient. There's a young woman I've been treating for a long time, with no success. Heal her and I'll publicly declare, here in this very place: 'Healers do exist and you are one of them.' "

The challenge might have been a trap, but I answered without pausing to consider:

"If your patient is not suffering from cancer or tuberculosis, I accept. Only I do not have my plants here and I stipulate that my treatment should be given under my personal supervision. I propose that I take her with me to Nice, where I will treat her free of charge and pay all her fares and expenses. I will bring her back in a month's time and you will be able to judge for yourself."

"Sir, the patient is my daughter. I accept your offer, only I will not allow you to pay her fares and expenses."

Everyone shouted and applauded, it was an extraordinary scene.

The young woman was called Yolande Bourla, and she was married to a shirt-maker in Bab-el-Oued. Her father, Doctor Timsit, explained to me that ever since the age of three she had suffered from inflammation of the spleen, but no one had ever been able to determine the cause. I began by relieving the violent pains which wracked her at times, applying to the region of the spleen a poultice based on round-leaved mallow and sage, which brought her almost immediate relief. Then, with my foot-baths, I set about treating her general state of health. She was in poor physical condition, for which milfoil, in conjunction with parsley, peppermint and thyme were the indicated remedy. For her nrves I chose single-seed hawthorn and poppy, and to restore her appetite I included some root of yellow gentian.

Three weeks later Yolande Bourla was no longer running

a temperature and she had gained eleven pounds (five kilos). The doctors from Paris who examined her declared that her spleen was perfectly healthy and functioning normally. When I went back with her to Algiers, her father and her husband kept exclaiming: "It's a miracle!" Doctor Timsit was determined to be true to his word and wanted to hire the cinema in order to hail me publicly as a healer, and I had some trouble in persuading him to do nothing of the kind.

This wasn't the first time a doctor had entrusted the health of his daughter to me, nor was it to be the last. Throughout all my years as a healer I have always been on the best of terms with doctors themselves, many of whom have addressed and treated me as a medical colleague. I have letters from many doctors thanking me warmly for healing members of their families. One eminent cancer specialist and high medical administrator wrote: "The name of Mességué will one day enter the annals of Science." A surgeon wrote warmly: ". . . I feel your charitable attitude is worthy of the highest medical tradition.

"I hope that all your efforts will not be in vain and that you will succeed where we have all failed.

"In any case I shall not fail to keep you informed of the results, and I sincerely hope for the success of what I consider an experiment in purely the best interests, and for the cure of our patient.

"In a case like this, when the most modern scientific and rational methods have demonstrated their utter powerlessness—methods I have not been the only one to apply, since this patient has twice spent a month in the dermatology unit of Professor N. in Lille—observation of empirical treatment and its eventual results can give us invaluable information and provide a source of fruitful knowledge. It is this that was in my mind when I brought you this patient.

"I thank you again for receiving us so kindly, and beg you, etc. etc."

It has very often happened that doctors, whom I would never dare call "colleagues," have sent patients to me asking me to draw up a true diagnosis of their case.

But my most important encouragement, the encouragement that really had a tremendous influence on my career, came from Doctor Claoué, who demonstrated his confidence in me the way he said:

"Maurice, I'd like you to see what you can do for some friends of mine, Lord and Lady X."

To treat Lord X would be tantamount to setting foot on the red carpet that led to the British Court. I couldn't help laughing to myself at the vision of a little Mességué like a tiny black dot on a long royal carpet leading to . . . the Queen of England. The childish notion appealed to me.

I very nearly lost my footing at the outset, by arriving one and a half minutes late for my appointment with Lord X at the Négresco.

I was confronted by a tall gentleman, six foot seven inches tall and about seventy years of age, with silver grey hair and a red carnation in his buttonhole, who was standing stiffly erect in the middle of his hotel suite and glaring at me severely:

"Sir, you must learn that an English lord is never kept waiting, as even the Queen knows."

It wasn't a very promising start. And I lost what little self-assurance still remained to me when Lady X entered. She was almost as tall as her husband, nearly six foot five, slim, very elegant. Between them I looked like a dwarf. He inspected me through his monocle and she through her lorgnette, conveying the impression that in their eyes I was some unknown species of insect. But my task has always been the saving of me in all kinds of situations. When I am considering treatment, nothing else matters, and I am no more impressed by a queen than by a washerwoman.

Lord X was dragging his leg noticeably. He had very bad arthritis of the hip. I knew that he was enduring great pain, and I admired him for the impassivity of his bearing, which allowed no trace of his suffering to show in his face.

"I will not ask if you are in pain, as an English Lord never feels pain! . . ."

Like a true Englishman, he appreciated my humor:

"Let's say that I'd like to be more agile than I am . . ."

"You will be."

"And you're going to manage it with that little contraption?"

He pointed to my pendulum.

"No, this is just my instrument for testing. Didn't Dr. Claoué tell you that I treat people with the plants we call medicinal?"

"He only told me that you're the man I need, and I trust his judgment."

A few moments later Lord X was offering me a whisky, a drink I loathe and which I politely refused. As I had been giving him some advice regarding his diet, he said:

"I imagine you don't allow this either?"

"For you I'd recommend your other national beverage, tea."

They very quickly became real friends of mine. Lady X was an amazing woman, coolly intelligent, at times tough, even cruelly witty. In social matters she could be quite ruthless. Towards me she was always extraordinarily kind.

Claoué had guessed rightly. A year later I was involved in my second court case (nor was it to be my last). I was to appear before the Bench roughly once a year for the next twenty years! Why? The procedure is quite simple and never varies: a doctor, frequently one with consulting rooms in the same block, notifies the Medical Council that someone is practicing medicine "illegally." The Council, generally in agreement with the professional associations, lays the matter before the public prosecutor and by bringing a civil action obliges him to take proceedings. It can happen that the public prosecutor takes proceedings of his own accord, but this has never occurred in my case.

This time I was not so shattered by the ordeal, but it was nevertheless extremely irritating. I have never been able to get used to these legal proceedings. For me they typify blind law with all its limitations, moving with a mechanical lack of discrimination.

My lawyer was again Mr. Pasquini, the future vice-president of the National Assembly. I had met him in Nice and taken to him at once. I was struck by his intelligence and his remarkable talent, he was young and handsome, with great personal magnetism and an aura of tremendous power. Just to see him smile had an immensely cheering effect. I was quite disturbed over the impending hearing and said:

"If they came and said: 'We're taking you to court because after four or five months of your treatment a patient is in such a bad way that the medical profession cannot save him." This would be something I could understand. But nobody ever mentions the patients when I'm taken to court. They're of no concern to anyone. Nobody complains that I make them better, that I cure them, or even harm them—their only complaint is that I practice medicine. The very existence of patients would never enter into it if I did not have to produce them as witnesses. But what the Medical Council never forgets to bring up is the matter of my "ill-gotten gains." I am criticized for taking payment, without regard to the number of patients I treat free of charge, who total more than a third of my clientele. When I produced letters of thanks to prove it, the Council's reply was:

"You have no right to treat people free of charge either . . ."

"My poor Maurice, you're sometimes really extraordinarily naïve. Have you thought that if you didn't cure your patients, that if you made just one single mistake, they'd be after you for manslaughter and as well as being fined, you'd run the risk of going to prison?"

I was furious and shouted:

"They're mad, they're criminal. It's not an action on behalf of public health that they're taking against me, it's an
action against my patients, and I'll tell them so. And don't
think you can stop me."

The more I shouted, the more Mr. Pasquini laughed.
But he was a bit worried all the same, for he knew, as do
all my friends, that when my wrath is aroused by something, I say so and I don't give a fig for the consequences.

The preliminary investigation of my second case was con-
ducted with great care and in deadly earnest. The police
inquiry could hardly have been stricter had I been accused
of being a second Boston Strangler. The amount of effort
they put into it was so disproportionate to the offense that
the effect became farcical. One morning, at the statutory
hour of sunrise, two police inspectors presented themselves
at my home in Porte Champerret.

"We are commissioned by the examining magistrate to
confirm the presence of clients in your house and to sub-
stantiate the charge. You are therefore requested in no way
to impede us in the performance of our duty."

Standing by the window, one of the inspectors watched
the street while the other watched the door.

By the end of the morning not a single patient had rung
my doorbell, and as the inspectors were sufficiently well-
informed to know that I normally see a great many, one of
them snapped at me suspiciously:

"So nobody is going to show up today? You've been tipped
off and you've cancelled your appointments."

He was quite right, I had in fact cancelled all my appointments for that day in order to be free for one particular
person. Contrary to what he was thinking, his presence,
along with that of his colleague, was quite acceptable, as
I might well have arranged for it myself as a security measure on behalf of the personnage I was expecting.

In an increasingly disagreeable tone, he continued: "We'll
wait as long as we have to, but we'll see your clients! . . ."

He was right again, for ten minutes later he could see

through the window a Rolls-Royce from the British Embassy drawing up outside my door. Lord X stepped out and bowed formally before a young woman prettily swathed in mink. I was waiting in the entrance hall to greet my client, whose appointment had been made by Lord X himself. I was about to open the door when the inspector leapt forward to do so. He gasped with astonishment. The young woman who entered was a charming and important member of the British royal family. That very morning her photograph had been in every newspaper in Paris.

The two panic-stricken police inspectors mumbled what was presumably some kind of apology and disappeared. Lord X has always thought that I'd called in the police for the protection of this royal personage.

Later, when I told Lady X about my impending court case, she looked long and steadily at me:

"It is a shocking thing that the law in your country should lead to this. Please make whatever arrangements are necessary for me to come and tell these magistrates what they ought to be told."

In the courtroom of the 16th court of summary jurisdiction in the Palais de Justice that month of July 1950, the atmosphere was stormy and oppressive. The hearing opened in a limp, almost indifferent mood, which did not please Mr. Pasquini. Indifference is the worst thing in court, for a sleepy courtroom is liable to pass the most unjust verdicts. The journalists were paying scarcely any attention when Mr. Pasquini placed some huge bundles of letters on the desk of the presiding judge, saying:

"There, Your Honor, are the testimonies of patients who have been unable to attend. There would hardly have been room for them anyway—there are two thousand!"

Mr. Pasquini had subpoenaed fifty-eight witnesses, but as the judge had decided to accord only sixty minutes to examination, it had barely been possible for fifteen witnesses to be heard. We were not in Nice now, where everything becomes theater, commedia dell'arte. Here there was no room for miracles and marvels, only for the law, strictly applied. A healer without a medical school diploma was a quack; I was beside myself with indignation.

The public started to warm up when some of the witnesses were examined. Mr. Glenna, with a fine southern accent which failed to bring any sunshine into the courtroom, declared:

"I am 100 percent disabled and in addition I kept getting lung abscesses: as fast as one would heal, another would return . . . The doctors had more than given me up. The last two doctors had told me there was no hope and my wife was already preparing to go into mourning when her sister, who lives in Nice, told her that Mr. Maurice was performing miracles with his plants. I believe in herbs, myself. He gave me poultices and foot-baths, and my doctor in Menton had to admit that I was cured. My doctor said that there are kinds of diseases for which the healers have cures which licensed medical men consider impossible. He even went in person to Mr. Mességué to tell him: 'I don't believe in you, but I must acknowledge the fact that you've saved this unlucky fellow!'

"The unlucky fellow was myself. Doctors are the kind of people who always have to be right. When you die they say: 'I said he would' and when you get better they say: 'I knew I wasn't wrong.' "

The courtroom was by now full of noise and applause and the judge threatened to have the place cleared.

Such humble testimonies did nothing to shake the scepticism of the Bench, nor did the testimonies of doctors.

My heart leaped when I heard the judge say:

"We have spent enough time on this. Call the last witness."

This was Lady X.

She made a memorable entrance.

Wearing elbow-length kid gloves, a muslin gown and a flowing cape, this tall Victorian lady looked more as if she belonged on the lawns of some garden party than in the fusty precincts of a courtroom. With a flick of the wrist she opened her lorgnette and looked at the presiding judge. She was respectfully accompanied by an English lawyer in pin-striped trousers and black jacket, his bowler hat, gloves and leather briefcase in his hand. These two personages had changed the atmosphere in a second.

At a sign from the judge, the usher had brought a chair for Lady X—an honor which in France is reserved only for ministers. She sat down with the same proud poise as in her own drawing-room.

"Please be so kind as to remove your gloves, Madam," the judge requested.

Her lawyer leaned attentively towards her and with quite obvious difficulty she very slowly unfastened the buttons of her long gloves.

The entire courtroom watched in silent fascination.

"Now," continued the judge, "raise your right hand and swear to tell the truth, say I swear . . ."

Lady X never even moved her hand but replied, succinctly:

"Members of our family, sir, always tell the truth!"

It was astonishing. She gave her evidence in the same tone.

"There is no point in your asking me questions, I know what I want to say. In our country to complain of private matters such as one's health is not done. I tell you this so that you will know that if I am here it is not to talk about myself but to defend a man for whom we have the highest regard.

"For many years I used to have what I believe you call migraines. There was nothing more our doctors could do for me. They had tried everything they knew. Mr. Mességué cured me. He is not a quack, as you say he is, he is a good, honest man.

"I love France and I am shocked to see Maurice Mességué brought before the courts of this country accused of being guilty of healing.

"I have nothing further to say."

She calmly buttoned up her gloves again, rose to her feet and with a curt nod towards the Bench left the courtroom.

I don't know if it did my case any good, but it certainly made me feel better.

I was sentenced to a fine of $16.00 with $120.00 damages, but this, in spite of my own remonstrances, did not prevent my patients from bearing me in triumph through the waiting hall.

16

Winston Churchill

Whenever i was at the Cap d'Aïl, I often saw Lord X, since we were neighbors. My little villa was surrounded by British Press Lords: on one side Lord X, and on the other; Lord Beaverbrook, who lived in the villa Capocina, a rococo palace built in the style of the coast's heyday, where Winston Churchill often stayed.

One evening Lord X said to me: "I must introduce you to one of your neighbors, I think you'll appreciate each other."

I thanked him, but there was nothing unusual about his suggestion. I owed my English clientele to the X family. Their acquaintances, or nearly all, had one foot in the court or the landed gentry. I had forgotten about this when one morning the telephone rang. I picked up the receiver and heard a deep voice with a marked English accent. I have a retentive ear, and I had the feeling this was a voice I'd heard before.

"Mr. Maurice Mességué?"

"Speaking."

"Winston Churchill here. I gather you're treating X. I'd like to see you. I don't need any treatment, I'm never ill, but I thought we might have a little talk about things, especially about what to do if you want to live to a ripe old age. I think it's time I gave the matter some thought."

He was already well over seventy.

"I'm at your service, Mr. President." Ever since I'd known Herriot, I called all great political figures "President." It was a sensible system because it saved me from getting their titles wrong, and, besides, there was a democratic touch about it that afforded me some satisfaction.

The next day, at the palatial Villa Capocina, a kind of major-domo greeted me: "Please come this way. Sir Winston Churchill is expecting you."

In a corner of the grounds, beneath the pine trees overlooking the sea, I saw the famous bulldog silhouette of Churchill. He was sitting at his easel and painting in strong colors the rocks and sea I had stared at so long the day before, when I had been thinking about him. He was wearing faded old dungarees, all covered with paint, a white felt Stetson to keep off the sun, with the legendary cigar stuck in the side of his mouth. When he saw me—he could see a great distance—he raised his hand in the familiar V salute, and the sight was so exactly as I had imagined it would be that I felt as if I were walking into a photograph from history.

At closer quarters, the colors on his canvas appeared even more violent.

"Do you like it?"

I thought his painting rather hideous, but I don't know how to tell a lie any more than I know how to pay a compliment. In this respect I suppose I still lack polish, but I don't like being rude or unkind, and so I said nothing.

"I see," said Churchill, mischievously screwing up his eyes, "that you don't dare to tell me it's—what do you say in French?—*moche*. Don't worry, though, the signature's worth something. I find painting very restful, because it means looking at just a very small part of the world, which is a lot less tiring than looking at a map of the whole thing.

"I told you, I'm as healthy as a baby. Have you noticed how all babies look like me? And d'you know why I look so rested? Because I can drop off to sleep anywhere at any time.

"I asked you to come so we could have a little chat about the future. It's my belief that life begins at eighty. Well, I'm seventy-nine now, so next year I'll have to think about getting seriously organized. X told me that even if your plants are old and dry, your ideas are fresh and new. What would you say, for example, if I told you I cough a lot?"

He was still painting, his eyes narrowed as he looked at the canvas, as if he attached no importance to my reply.

"Are you familiar with plants, Mr. President?"

"I'm familiar enough with the ones put on my dinner plate. As for the others, I'm not sure I've even seen them all. There's not much plant life at Ten Downing Street."

"For coughs, phytotherapists use plants that are good on your plate too—garlic, cabbage, cress, onion, thyme, marjoram and mint—as well as plants that look good in a vase: poppy, mallow, violets. There are also the wild flowers: borage, common flax, and great mullein, or Aaron's rod."

He turned to face me, joyfully sucking at his unlighted cigar:

"You didn't say: stop smoking. You're cleverer than a doctor! And will you settle my cough with all these plants?"

"No, I'll mix a simpler cocktail, but I'll certainly include mallow. It's a plant I'm very fond of and it can be used all year round. When the flowers are finished you take the leaves, and when the leaves have dropped you use the root. You'll be pleased to know it's often put in babies' bottles to soothe their coughs, and as a historian, sir, you'll be interested to know that the Ancient Romans used to eat young mallow shoots both cooked and in salads. Cicero mentions it in his letters, and Horace has a line in one of his odes: olives, chicory and light mallow . . ."

"Don't let that fool you, the Romans fed themselves on good meat, not herbs."

"And for you I'd also include violet."

Churchill roared with laughter.

"That's a flower that goes very well with my modesty."

"Don't laugh, Sir, it will be very good for your cough."

I liked Winston Churchill from the first. He was a man with an extraordinary, overwhelming personality, and I was completely won over by his simplicity, his outspokenness, his humor, and his way of taking himself seriously and at the same time making fun of himself. We were soon on familiar terms, and I even invited him round for lunch.

"I hope," he said when he arrived, "that we're going to eat plenty of herbs that are good for the health."

"Mushrooms in garlic, our local cassoulet and all the trimmings, potted goose from the Gers, and Toulouse sausages. Roquefort, cherry tart, and a fine, full-bodied Bergerac."

We finished with an old Armagnac.

"Taste it, Mr. President. It has an aroma of violets."

"That's why it's good for me."

Churchill's eyes were moist with the affection of a gourmand for good food, and his cheeks were like two little round apples. I had never seen his nose look so small or his smile so broad.

"Mességué, they've slandered you. That joker X told me that your diet was wretched and made a man irritable. Either he's very hard to please, or you're like every other doctor. They all say: 'Do what I tell you, but don't do what I do.'"

Winston Churchill was not very fond of doctors. It was he who taught me the only English proverb I know: "An apple a day keeps the doctor away," to which he added his own ending, "especially if you're a good shot!" Speaking of Lord Moran, his personal physician, he told me: "He's marvelous, he really works very hard at the job of poisoning your life in order to save it. Thanks to him I know what I'll die of: boredom."

Churchill's humor was often quite scathing and merciless, which perhaps explains why Lord Moran, after the death of his patient, wrote such merciless memoirs about him.

I managed to lecture him all the same. Whenever he was in a good mood, which was frequently, I would take advantage of it and tell him:

"You should follow my example, Mr. President. I don't drink, I don't smoke, I eat sensibly, and I do a lot of walking. This is why I'm in good health."

"It's when you're my age that I'll be able to judge if your regimen was really good. And if I'm still around to judge, you'll have to admit that mine was better! It's simple: I smoke, I drink, I never take any exercise, and my health's every bit as good as yours. You know why? The germs are either stupefied with sleep, asphyxiated by smoke or killed by alcohol."

And he gave one of those secret chuckles of his, crinkling up his eyes.

"That's not altogether the truth, of course, Mességué, and you're a good enough chap for me to admit that these days I'm really being very good. I hardly smoke at all, to my regret. People keep on giving me masses of cigars, all from Davidoff, who's been my supplier for half a century. Ah, if I could only live long enough to smoke them all! I ration myself, but you mustn't tell anyone. People must still see their ageing Lion tearing up his gazelle, or they'd say he's lost his teeth. In public you're always on show, so I always have a glass at my fingertips and a 'Winston Churchill' [1] between my lips. But the glass remains full and I let the cigar go out. I've even got a good trick for photographers waiting at airports. I always keep a half-smoked cigar on me and produce it just as we land. I spend the rest of the journey sucking sweets. I'll choose violet-scented ones now, because of you. But I couldn't tell that to the

[1] Brand of cigar created in homage to Churchill. They can still be found in Belgium.

journalists; they're not like you—they'd rather see me with a cigar."

Churchill had a very real affection for journalists, even though he gave them a hard time. One afternoon I heard a young reporter, who had obtained permission to interview him on the Cap d'Ail, say to Churchill, hoping to please him, "Sir, I hope I'll be able to interview you again on your hundredth birthday."

Churchill, rolling the cigar between his lips so that it was pointing like a piece of artillery at the sky, replied, "I don't see why not, you seem quite young and you look fit enough."

He liked to recall that journalism had once been his own profession: "I was a war correspondent in Cuba (in the Spanish-American War). The pay was rotten, but I have very pleasant memories. You really could get Havanas for next to nothing there."

I treated Churchill from 1950 to 1957, or perhaps I should say I chatted with him on and off for seven years. For he didn't take his treatments at all seriously. As soon as he felt the slightest improvement he would give up. However, he didn't deny the virtues of my herbs, and besides, he had an open mind. Confronted with anything that might have seemed odd, he always said: "Just because you can't explain a thing is no reason to deny it."

While he was staying in Marrakesh he had had himself treated by a mesmerist named Vallier.

"I can't explain why, but I assure you that when that mesmerist passed his hands over me I felt a new flow of energy and a tightening of the muscles."

To me the most extraordinary thing about Winston Churchill was his friendship and fidelity. He never came to the Cap d'Ail without telephoning me. There were two things about me that he valued: I didn't bother him and I was full of fight. He was amused by the fact that I kept getting prosecuted, and he despised people who think that the way to treat an insult is to ignore it.

"It's stupid, Mességué. The only answer to an insult is an insult, and if that isn't enough, then a slap in the face or a good hard punch. You don't defend your honor by sitting on it!"

He fostered his reputation as a man who didn't mince words, because it allowed him to say what he thought. One day, at a grand dinner I was also attending, Churchill overheard the end of a sentence: ". . . the Liberation of France was terrible." Chewing on his cigar and looking deliberately blank, he broke in with: "In England we didn't have the same problems."

"And if you'd been in de Gaulle's shoes, what would you have done?"

"I'd have taken Marshal Pétain by the hand and together we'd have walked up the Champs-Elysées."

Then he added: "But I am only a guest here, I have no right to give an opinion."

It was surprising to discover that two such different men as Edouard Herriot and Winston Churchill should have an almost identical opinion on the Pétain–de Gaulle issue.

Churchill had been very fond of Roosevelt, and the two men had got on very well together. When he spoke of him, he would say: "That was a good man, a fine man, and his outlook was first-rate. Only at Yalta he wasn't the same man any more; you could tell he was very ill. When a man has to struggle against his own body he has less strength for struggling against other people. It was very hard standing up to Stalin. That man had the look of a madman, and when he was talking he'd stare at you with those cruel, inhuman eyes of his. He had a strange face—as though the halves of two different faces had been joined together. Beneath that fatherly great moustache his lips would be smiling, and above it were those hypnotic, almost fixed, soulless eyes. Only I'm not the person to be so easily hypnotized, I resist that kind of influence very well. His power lay in having no heart, no feeling of any kind, and Roosevelt was a bit frightened by this total lack of humanity."

Winston Churchill was a man I greatly admired. Even when he began to have difficulty in getting about, his mind was as agile as ever, although he took his time when speaking. Behind that bulldog exterior was a highly sensitive, highly sentimental, highly vulnerable man. You could easily hurt him, and—unexpectedly in a man of such strength, a man who was Prime Minister and one of the best-loved men in the world—as soon as he found himself in the company of a woman he was completely disarmed.

Towards his wife, this rough, pugnacious and at times aggressive man behaved with surprising gentleness and delicacy. He would talk to me about her for hours.

"Lady Clementine, Mességué, was the most famous beauty in England, and look at her, isn't she still the most beautiful of the older, charming ladies?"

It was true.

Their love had endured for fifty years, and if he inadvertently showed her any disrespect he was wretched. Churchill didn't like being interrupted when he was telling a story, and he could be very loquacious. One day I happened to be standing next to him at the préfecture in Strasbourg, and while he was telling some anecdote his wife was chatting with someone else. He broke off and said: "Shut up, please!" and then, covered in confusion, he immediately went to her and kissed her hand. "I am very sorry, darling."

"The only quarrel I ever had with Clemmie," he told me once, "was over an old car. We had this ancient yellow Austin that I was very fond of, but I think she was rather ashamed to be seen in it. So one day she sold it for $112.00. When I found out I was furious and went straight to the garage to buy it back. I asked, 'How much do you want for this old heap?'—thinking I was being crafty by disparaging it."

"$280.00, sir."

"But that's twice what it cost!"

"It's half of what it's worth, sir; it belonged to the Prime Minister!"

"So I bought back my own car—the one time in my life I ever made a business deal. The incident led me to conclude that I'd been right not to go into commerce."

The death of Winston Churchill grieved me deeply. For the first and only time in my life, I, who sent only red roses, wanted him to have violets. On television I followed the long funeral procession and shared the mourning that hung like a shroud over England. In my imagination, I could see my bunch of violets and hear Churchill asking, roguishly as ever:

"Mességué, do you think I need violets to get me to sing with the angels?"

17

Robert Schuman
and Konrad Adenauer

MEN ARE LIKE PLANTS. They have their good qualities and their bad. Even the best of my good herbs can become dangerous and harmful. Roman camomile, for example, that family panacea with such a good name for aiding the digestion and settling a nervous stomach, can cause vomiting if taken in too large doses. Linden blossoms, which so effectively induce sleep, can cause insomnia if the doses are too strong. Even the greater celandine, which I value so highly, is so toxic that if very strong doses are ingested it can be fatal. I feel the same curiosity, and the same affection for men and all growing things. This helps me greatly in my treatments.

Whenever someone came to my father, he would say: "Let yourself go. Tell me first if there's anything wrong at home."

And with the extraordinary patience of a man with all the time in the world to spare, he would listen to his patient complaining about his life and his body, often both at once.

"You see, *mon chéri,*" he used to say to me, "a man's life and his body go together, they travel the same road. Each affects the other, so to treat the one you have to know the other." Our country doctors used to proceed in the same fashion, treating a man's worries at the same time as his liver.

It has been the plain common sense I inherited from my father that has saved me from taking myself too seriously. In barely four years I had gone from poverty to wealth. One day a hall-porter was threatening to kick me out of his hotel, and the next—or so it seemed—I was being fussed over by people I'd never even have dreamed of approaching. It had all been enough to turn even the most level head. There had been times when I felt my head swelling up like a balloon; it was hard to remain unaffected by incidents such as this:

I was in Marrakesh to give a lecture, when two young men came to see me at the Mamounia, where I was staying. They were Moroccans in European dress, very elegant and very courteous, in fact a perfect combination of Arabian good manners and European education.

"Sir, we were at your lecture and we'd like you to come and see our father."

"Gentlemen, I'm very sorry, but I can't. I never give consultations in a town where I'm invited to speak."

Knowing the customs of the country, I offered them a coffee. With great delicacy they let me know that they were ready to pay me a million francs if I accepted.

"No, I can't. In no circumstances could I accept. It's a matter of principle. I'm sure you'll understand."

They rose, said good-bye and departed. The next morning, at seven o'clock, the hotel switchboard operator called me: "General X, the town mayor, would like to see you."

I couldn't imagine why, but I told her to send him up. In due course a general in a fine uniform entered my room and clicked his heels: "Sir, I pay you my respects."

I was thirty years old and a general was paying me his respects—me, a plain private. This was amazing enough, and I was thoroughly enjoying the humor of it, but there was even better to come.

"Sir, yesterday you spoke to the sons of His Excellency, El Glaoui, Pasha of Marrakesh, and I am told that you refused to go and see their father. El Glaoui has telephoned the President, who has instructed me to ask you if you will kindly accede to His Excellency's wishes."

This was staggering. A general was asking me in the name of the Government to practice the kind of healing for which in France I was harried and prosecuted.

I think I am one of very few Europeans to have entered the bedchamber of El Glaoui—a bedchamber out of an Arabian fairy tale—where I first saw that tall, thin, distinguished old man with the noble bearing of a real ruler. He believed in the virtues of my plants, and I put them at his disposal.

In such a situation, it is difficult not to have a moment of vanity, but I say to myself: You're only a peasant, the son of Camille, and that brings me back to reality at once. Another thing has helped me: Among all these famous people, I have been lucky to meet men who were not merely celebrities but human beings of stature, whose modesty has been a priceless example to me. The man who perhaps influenced me the most in this respect was Robert Schuman.

One morning when I had been to see Herriot, he said to me: "Maurice, I want you to meet one of my best friends. We don't always see eye to eye, especially over your Good Lord, but to my mind the man is a saint. It's Robert Schuman."

He had made an appointment for me, and I made my way to the rue du Bac, where Schuman lived in a little three-room apartment. I don't remember having much curiosity about meeting him, or even thinking about it particularly, nor did I have a clear picture of his physical appearance. I had seen newspaper photographs and probably one or two caricatures, and had gathered that he wasn't very prepossessing in appearance.

When Marie, his "Césarine," opened the door to me, I thought I must have come to the wrong floor. His apartment was more like the lodgings of an impoverished churchman than the home of a political figure. In his office there was a prie-dieu, to which pious hands had imparted a patina, and humble knees had bequeathed lumps and hollows. On the wall hung an uncompromising plain black crucifix, and in a basin of holy water was some greenery from the last Palm Sunday. The only piece of furniture that could be called comfortable was in the bedroom—a country-parson armchair upholstered in green velvet, with a crocheted antimacassar, although I've never been sure that Schuman ever actually dared sit in it.

I remember my first meeting with him very clearly. He was standing very erect, wearing a suit of some thick grey stuff, and stout black shoes with rounded toes. In all the fourteen years I knew him I never saw him wear any other kind—and he gave an immediate impression of quite astonishing ugliness. He had a small, bald head like a plucked bird, elephantine ears and a long giraffe neck on an ungainly body. My father would have said he was "as long as a day without bread."

"How do you like my bachelor pad?"

The inappropriateness of the description evidently tickled his sense of humor, for behind his spectacles, I discerned a roguish twinkle that I was soon to learn to enjoy.

"I call it that because, after all, I am an old bachelor. Mr. Mességué. I have never been married, and I wear long underpants, as you'll be able to tell when you examine me."

His rugged Alsace accent sounded strange to my Gascon ear, more accustomed as I was to the lilting accents of the South. I started to ask him a few professional questions, examining him meanwhile. His grey complexion, colorless lips and dry hands with pale nails all denoted the mortification of the flesh and the meditations of the mind. If he was suffering from anything, it could only be the stomach. He looked at first sight so sad and austere that one might have taken him for a cold man, but his smile radiated goodness and tolerance. I never once heard him speak unkindly of anyone. He intrigued me. How on earth had this quiet, withdrawn man ever come to choose a career in politics, which favors the highwayman more than the monk? As soon as we were sufficiently good friends—which didn't take long—I asked him about it.

"People often ask me why I never married, and my answer to this answers your own question. When I was first elected deputy, in 1919, I married politics. Politics has been a real wife to me—demanding, often inconstant, but I am faithful for both of us. There are men who can devote themselves to a wife and to their profession, but I am not one of them. I'd always be afraid of injuring one to the detriment of the other. Why did I choose politics? From vanity, because I thought I might be able to make a useful contribution. And because I needed to devote myself to something, since I wasn't devoting myself to any one person."

It was becoming clear: he had taken up politics much as other men take holy orders. He knew himself well, for he would certainly have felt he owed a wife the kind of allegiance that would have complicated his professional life. He was scrupulously respectful of others, and couldn't bear to be a nuisance to anyone. One night, for example, he returned home from a sitting at the National Assembly, which had gone on until three in the morning, only to find that he had forgotten his keys.

What could I do, Mességué? Ring the doorbell and wake Marie? It was out of the question; she'd been working all day and she had a right to her night's sleep. So I sat on the stairs and waited until seven o'clock."

I could see him, perched neatly on the stairs like a shivering bird, waiting for Marie to wake up. Never for a moment did it enter his mind that his own sleep was more important than his housekeeper's. The episode was typical of Schuman, and taught me a great lesson in humility.

I've never had a patient so docile and so respectful of my advice, nor one so difficult to treat. I had chosen for him a preparation based on mallow, which was straightforward enough, but how was one to set about simplifying the diet of a man who doesn't even drink wine? Who doesn't eat anything except minced steak and boiled potatoes? Whose only stimulant is mint tea, and even that only on special occasions? Whose holidays are spent at the abbey of Ligugé in the Vienne?

Schuman's private life was a block of flawless crystal, and he was as scrupulous and honest towards the State as he was in everything else. One morning I remember seeing him quietly leave a first-class compartment of a train after a trip abroad.

"You must be very tired, why didn't you take a sleeping car?" I asked him.

"France has better things to do with her money than spend it on that kind of thing. One can sleep quite well sitting up," but I knew this wasn't true, for he had trouble in sleeping.

He administered State affairs as he would his own, and he was so economical that every evening, at the Ministry, he would go round after his colleagues had left, switching off all the lights.

"I'm a bit like Georges Clémenceau," he would say: "First to come and last to leave. Have you heard about the day Clémenceau was made President of the Council? I believe it's a true story. Apparently Clémenceau, followed by his colleagues, was making an official tour of the building at about eleven-thirty in the morning. They entered the first office, but there was no one there. Then they looked in the second, third, fourth—all empty. Finally in the fifth they found a draughtsman quietly sleeping at his desk, his head pillowed on his arms.

"A zealous young secretary sprang forward to waken him, but 'the Tiger' stopped him. 'No, don't wake him up, he might go!' "

It was through Schuman that I came to love Alsace. In fact, he made me a Gascon Alsatian. I had always said, "A man has two countries, his homeland and his village," but now I say, "He has three: his homeland, his village and Alsace." I am tremendously fond of the Alsatians, who are serious, hard-working, sensitive and cheerful people.

Schuman's great concept, as everyone knows, was a Federated Europe, but he never envisaged this without the real participation of Germany. For hours we would walk along side by side with the slow plodding pace of two peasants, tramping the rich, fertile soil of Alsace as Schuman quietly built up that new world of his, picking his words with care and thought.

"Mr. Mességué"—he always called me "Mister"—"we must win the war quickly" (this was his obsession). "We must make war impossible. For that to be so we must have a Federated Europe. We are the nut between the jaws of the nutcracker: the USA and the USSR. But our Europe must include West Germany, before the reunification of the two Germanies, which will sooner or later take place. They're a serious, hard-working nation in peacetime, tough and dangerous in war. It's better to be their friends. The Germans know the cost of every gesture, of every nail that's hammered in, of every brick that's laid. Europe can't do without them. Realists, who see things before other people do, are always called utopians. But I don't mind, I shall go on fighting for this concept as long as I have to."

I had grown so attached to Alsace, far though it was from my own part of the country, that I had rented a hunting preserve at Marckolsheim. I often went with Schuman to Strasbourg when he was lecturing on Europe. He was a very poor speaker. Lacking confidence in himself, he always read from a prepared text, but his reading was even worse than when he spoke extemporaneously.

One evening when he was giving a lecture to the Strasbourg Officers' Club, a young woman in the front row—a splendid young woman, beautiful as a goddess, her blonde hair becomingly tied in a pony tail, which was then the latest fashion—stood up and shouted: "Oh, shut up, you old fool!"

Schuman unhurriedly raised his spectacles in that familiar way of his and looked at the young woman: "Oh, Mademoiselle, such ugly words in such a pretty mouth!"

That did it. The students who had come with the intention of heckling him—for his ideas were still not very popular—listened attentively to the end and even applauded him. Once he had captured the attention of his audience, this unassuming, self-effacing man could convey a faith and an honesty that were very convincing.

I was at my place at Marckolsheim when he said to me one day: "Mr. Mességué, I want you to meet a colleague and friend of mine. He also treats people with plants, like yourself."

I assumed he meant a German competitor in my own field, which was fine by me. In any case, Schuman had never asked me for anything. If he wanted me to meet this man, I knew it must be for a reason.

"Delighted. Bring your friend along tomorrow morning. I'll organize a beat for him."

"But he doesn't shoot any more than I do."

"Is he fond of walking?"

"As much as I am."

"Fine, then perhaps you'll both be my beaters?"

"That will be great fun, you've no idea. We'll see you tomorrow then."

From the way Schuman's eyes were twinkling behind his spectacles, I should have been on my guard and realized that he had a surprise up his sleeve. He certainly had—a big one.

The next day was lovely: the late autumn mist, pale with sunshine, hung in tendrils like silken hair among the branches of the fir trees. The dogs were straining impatiently at the leash, car doors were slamming cheerfully, we were all gathering for the day's shooting, happily stamping our feet on the road. I was waiting for Schuman to arrive to give the signal to start when I saw a Mercedes pulling up some distance away. The features of his "col-

league and friend" were blurred by the mist, but his silhouette was unmistakably German: Tyrolean felt hat with bad-
ger-hair feather, green loden-cape, plus-fours, thick natural-
wool socks and stout hunting shoes. His face struck me
as rather flat and featureless, and then suddenly I recognized him: Chancellor Konrad Adenauer, the oldest states-
man of Europe, and ranking with Churchill and de Gaulle
as one of the most illustrious.

I really hadn't been expecting this, and my guests, of
course, were even more astounded than I was. He looked
at me with those cold, authoritarian eyes of his and, speaking in rather poor French with a harsh guttural accent,
said:

"Mr. Mességué, you are a colleague of mine." He stressed
the word colleague. "We share the same belief. That's
something that brings men"—glancing at Schuman who was
observing us from behind his spectacles—"and nations together. Only, as a healer, you're out of luck with me. I
treat myself with my own plants, and the Federal German
State is very generous too. I'm allocated three official doctors. So, you can see, I'm well taken care of, and I'm afraid
my doctors wouldn't stand for it if I consulted you." He
chuckled. "They'd be afraid you might become a kind of
French Rasputin! But we can talk later. Since we're here
for the shooting, let's go!"

I remember very clearly that day spent out in the open.
All morning the Federal Chancellor and Robert Schuman
tramped with evident enjoyment over ground covered with
moss and smooth brown pine needles and thick with
bushes, joyfully beating the undergrowth to flush a fat
brown capuchin pigeon or a pheasant. I think I may be the
only man in Europe who ever went shooting with the Chancellor as his beater.

It wasn't from any lack of consideration for my guest
that I didn't at once abandon the day's shooting. I very
much wanted to see this stiff and unbending Chancellor relax in the countryside. I wanted to observe him and form

my own impressions, and as a result, I shot very badly that day. The man impressed me. He was as unaffected in his Bavarian clothes as Schuman in his grey suit, but there was no softening in his expression. He was unlike Herriot or Churchill, for he lacked the good nature of the former and the humor of the latter. His reputation as an "old fox" was of long standing and I thought it a good assessment. With Adenauer I wasn't at ease, and therefore far from my best. I feel free to be myself only in the warmth of sympathy and friendliness. That was how it was that day, and yet I was immensely curious about the man who walked beside me. I wondered what he was hiding behind that scarred, flattened face, the mask that was the result of a car accident in 1917.

The pale sunshine filtering through the pine trees lent the forest something of the feeling of a cathedral. It was very beautiful but lofty. Shortly before midday I abandoned my gun and we went on walking.

Adenauer had kept his stick, and from time to time he would gently scratch the soil to uncover a mushroom or a small plant, a gesture that made me feel more at home with him. The truth is that there was a great distance between us—myself a lad from the Gers, and he the Chancellor of Germany. Nearly half a century divided us, for I was then thirty and he was seventy-seven. He gently tapped a stem of cranberry.

"*Preiselbeere.*"

"Cranberry," Schuman translated.

"What do you use them for, Mr. Mességué?"

"Nothing, Mr. President. There aren't any in the Gers where I come from and I use only the plants that grow locally, the plants my family has tested for generations."

"I see. Well, it has the same qualities as this," pointing to the black bilberries.

"The red ones are more astringent, more acid, and sometimes harder for a sensitive stomach to tolerate."

Conversation between us was rather halting, for we used

a mixture of French and German, and Schuman had to act as interpreter.

"You know, I have a great belief in plants. These *Preiselbeeren* are good for dysentery, for example, and the leaves are a well-known anti-diabetic. They're also very effective against infections of the urinary system, and they can be used as a gargle for a sore throat. What do you use for all these things?"

"Bramble leaves for dysentery and heather for urinary infections."

"So you need two plants; we need only one. And I haven't finished: the fruit is rich in sugar and vitamins A and C and minerals. As a tincture we use it for thrush, stomatitis, buccal psoriasis, tonsilitis and eczema."

He stopped and looked at me, and I didn't dare to tell him that in France we are familiar with the various uses of red bilberries, even though I personally do not use them. I felt as if I were taking some examination, and was feeling daunted at the prospect of the rest of the day.

"And do you use horseradish?"

"No, Mr. President, but did you know that we call it German mustard?"

For the first time I saw him smile, so I pressed on: "I can also tell you that horseradish is anti-scorbutic, stimulant, diuretic, expectorant, and, when applied directly to the skin, it acts as a counter-irritant. It is also a very good tonic, and is recommended in the treatment of scrofulous conditions, chlorosis, anemia debility and rickets. For horseradish, which doesn't exist in my country, I substitute watercress, which has exactly the same properties and the advantage of being less strong and therefore more easily tolerated by delicate stomachs."

"I can see you are very knowledgeable, Mr. Mességué. Do you know this Swedish recipe, which is really very good for rheumatism and all kinds of dropsy? You grate some horseradish root, moisten it with a little vinegar water and pour on some boiled milk. When the milk has curdled you collect the whey and drink one or two small glassfuls every day. Personally I prefer grated horseradish mixed with butter and spread on a slice of bread. It does you good and it tastes good."

"You can do that with watercress too."

"I'll try it. Prevention is better than cure, as the saying goes. My own weak point is my stomach." He turned to Schuman. "I think our job's responsible, don't you? So I've eaten oatmeal every morning for sixty years now. It's a very good safeguard against ulcers, and also a very good treatment for them. The French are very careless about their health; they start the day by drinking a poison: coffee with milk. As soon as they wake up, they overstimulate an empty stomach and tire their liver. What's your opinion?"

"Exactly the same as yours, Mr. President, but in the country, people are wiser. Most of our peasants have soup first thing in the morning."

We rejoined my other guests for a light lunch, not one of those huge meals that knocks you out and undoes all the good a day out shooting can do you. Although Adenauer didn't drink spirits, he enjoyed a glass of Rhine wine with his meals. It was his pet indulgence, and he was sent as many bottles as Churchill received cigars. After our snack, someone asked him:

"Does smoking bother you, Herr Kanzler?"

"I don't know. Nobody has ever smoked in front of me."

"Mr. Mességué, can you play *pétanque?*"

This was unexpected. He had apparently discovered the game when he was staying once in the south of France, and ever since then he had kept a set of bowls in his car. So we had a game there and then, and although his aim was better than his shot, he certainly knew how to play.

I was beginning to like the man, and with a single question he won me over completely.

"Do you like roses?"

"I love them. I can't live without them and it really hurts me to cut one. Sentimentally, red roses are my favorites, because they're the symbol of passion. According to legend, roses were once all white, until at a banquet of the gods, Cupid, who was hovering around Venus, upset an amphora of wine with his wing and it stained the roses red. Another version says that he pricked himself with a thorn and his blood stained the rose he was offering to Venus."

"Ach! You French, you're never serious! You mingle sentiment with everything!"

"Especially us Gascons, Mr. President. I think that red roses are the best, medicinally the most effective."

"For what reason?"

"The red rose of Provins is the only one to be used medicinally since it was brought back from the Crusades, so they say, by Thibaut de Champagne. It's stronger, richer in tannin."

"Perhaps, but pale roses and yellow roses have laxative properties that yours don't. But I'll grant you one thing. In the thirteenth century a German, Dr. Kruger, cured himself of phthisis with a 'conserve' of red roses. I must add that he completed his treatment with barley water. What do you use your roses for?"

"Intestinal disturbances, leukorrhea, hemorrhages, migraines of ophthalmic origin, and especially for coughs. It's an excellent expectorant."

"I prefer yellow roses; they are just as effective, I use them a great deal. I easily develop a cough, and I find yellow roses sweeter than red ones."

Later, Schuman informed me: "What the Chancellor didn't tell you is that he has a magnificent rose garden at Rhoendorf, his property in the Rhineland. Knowing his predilection for yellow roses, the growers have created a very beautiful sulphur-colored rose for him, and named it the 'Konrad Adenauer.'"

It would be fatuous of me to think that I could have influenced the Chancellor, but he showed great interest in my methods of gathering plants, and particularly in the fact that I use only plants that have been growing wild, and that I refuse to grow them on cultivated soil and force them with fertilizer. "That's good, that's excellent!" he kept saying. He also wanted to know whether I used barley and corn.

"I highly recommend both, but once again I stress the conditions under which they have been grown, since to me this is crucial."

"That's the problem with everything we eat today, Mr. Mességué. Our foodstuffs are no longer natural and wholesome."

He seemed sorry that he was powerless to change things.

"I think as you do, but I am also Head of State and I have to be mindful of the fact that Germany's economic position in the chemical industry is very important. At times I deplore certain aspects of our expansion in this field, but I console myself by remembering that chemistry also discovered aspirin."

We didn't actually exchange any "prescriptions," but we discussed at length the ways in which we used plants. He was particularly keen on infusions, and drank a great deal of barley water. "I always drink my little infusion last thing at night," he told me. Barley was his own magic plant, but he also made frequent use of maize stigma, sage and mallow. These were his favorite plants, but he had extensive knowledge of all plants and had tried a great many. Our meeting was a meeting of "professionals." I gave him some of my own ideas and he said he would try them, but I can't be sure that he ever did. Besides, he wasn't ill. He clearly had an iron constitution, or, as Schuman so aptly put it, "He's as tough as Kehl bridge."

The sun was about to set, dipping down behind the Black Forest—the Chancellor's forest—when he said:

"Look at me, Mr. Mességué. When I was twenty I was declared unfit for military service because of my lungs. When I was forty an insurance company turned down my application for a policy because they didn't think I'd last the year. And now, thirty years later, I work ten hours a day in my office, I travel, I inaugurate, I visit, I cover miles and miles, and when I get home I can still run up the fifty-four steps to my villa like a young man. I owe it all to plants, to nature. And all the husbands in Germany hate me because they daren't let their wives hear them complain that they're tired, for the wives only say: 'How do you suppose the Chancellor manages, at his age?' "

This wasn't the same man who had emerged from his car that morning looking so stern and suspicious. He was completely relaxed now, and warming to his subject:

"Tell me, what is age, after all? We call anyone an old man who's ten years older than we are. So we're always an old man to someone." Then, with an unexpected lack of inhibition, the Chancellor went on to talk about the question of virility, "which is very important to a man's equilibrium, and what really keeps a man young. So it's a good thing to take care of it, by massaging the base of the spine with an ointment made from brambles, hawthorn berries and mint. What's your own recipe?"

"Cow-parsley, greater celandine, mint and fenugreek."

Adenauer listened with interest, but I no more influenced him than he influenced me. As has so often been said of France and Germany, "We maintained our respective positions."

18

Impotence and Frigidity

SEXUAL PROBLEMS can arise at any age, and often most unexpectedly.

Prince Ali Khan had asked me to come and see him without telling me exactly what was the trouble, but from the way he had said on the telephone, "We'll talk about it man to man," I imagined it would be something of a "personal" nature. This didn't worry me, since I always get very good results—a success rate of 80 percent—in such cases.

Ali Khan's apartment in the Avenue de Madrid could best be described as sumptuous, furnished with a cheerful medley of eighteenth-century chests of drawers and Oriental rugs and carpets in dark reds and deep violet, the color of convolvulus minor. The statues, vases, bas-reliefs and modern paintings would have made a welcome addition to the Louvre.

Walking across these carpets I felt that I was walking in another world, so far removed were they from the big, worn red tiles of our kitchen in Gavarret. Yet I was not intimidated by the magnificent, unfamiliar décor. On such occasions I bear in mind that the millionaire or prince who has sent for me is a patient requiring treatment. This puts me sufficiently at ease, prepared to be surprised or shocked by nothing.

That day I needed all my calm and confidence when the

prince's valet showed me into his private suite. The prince was seated in an armchair, one hand resting in the hand of a manicurist, and surrounded by beautiful women. He greeted me with:

"Are you the fellow with the herbs? But you're young. That's funny. Because of your foot-baths I'd been expecting some wacky old man."

His vocabulary was often coarse, but his good breeding made it acceptable. I looked at him. The condition of his hair and his skin and the color of his nails all indicated a man in perfect health. He carelessly dismissed the manicurist, but the other young women were still flitting back and forth, and from time to time one of them would bend over him to ask about something or hand him a paper or whisper the name of whoever was on the telephone. I found it hard to remember that I was only a stone's throw from the Place de l'Etoile and not in some Oriental palace.

I had taken out my pendulum and was passing it over my patient.

"D'you believe in all this crap? You don't have to put on a show for me, you know."

He gave me an ironical, almost cynical smile, and there was a gentleness in his look that must have played havoc with women.

"Well, Mességué, how do you find me?"

"In perfect health."

"Yes, I smoke, I drink, I deny myself nothing. I indulge myself in whatever I fancy—only there's one 'but.' I know you've had a lot to do with sexual problems and you've been to places like Kuwait and certain Arab states, where they set great store by virility. They tell me you get very good results, and that after you've been there the women have no more complaints about their husbands. That's why I've sent for you. Let's say I've lost my appetite for love-making."

In simple and quite uninhibited terms, the prince told me that while his actual performance was unaffected, and he

indeed was still in full control of the act and its culmina-
tion, yet he found he was doing it more for the sake of
his health than from any real desire.

"It's getting me down, you understand. Does this lack of
interest in women around me mean that I'm growing old
before my time? Can you do anything for me?"

"Let me first ask you something: How many times a
week?"

He looked rather surprised.

"Three times a day regularly."

"And always successfully? Never any trouble?"

"Absolutely."

"Then, Prince, I think I ought to be consulting you!"

He laughed heartily, and I didn't see him again. On my
way home I reflected that it was certainly the first time I'd
ever been able to laugh at a sexual problem. On the contrary, I always took such matters very seriously, for they
can be quite tragic, and I am fully aware of their importance
to both men and women.

It is in sexual fulfillment that a couple find their personal
harmony and their happiness. I've had a lot to do with
this problem, for I have treated some fifteen thousand patients, achieving results varying from good to perfect with
rather more than twelve thousand of these patients. Despite
the current wave of eroticism and all the fine talk about
sexual freedom and education, sex is not a subject people
can always talk about easily and frankly. The French, who
are considered abroad as a pleasure-loving nation, find it
even harder to discuss sex than foreigners do. Only very
rarely does anyone tell me straight out that they have come
to see me because they can't make love, or because it gives
them no pleasure and is just a drag. I have to flush the truth
out of the tangled undergrowth of their complexes, like
flushing a frightened hare out of the bushes. I do not do
this from any taste for personal confidences, but because I
know full well the importance of sexual harmony to a person's general state of health, and particularly how it can

affect certain conditions, which to the patient might seem unrelated, such as duodenal ulcers, liver troubles, and nervous and even intestinal disorders.

Men keep silent because vanity makes it hard for a man to confess a lack of virility to another. The many women still conditioned by an upbringing that kept sex in the background are too shy or embarrassed to speak of it. There are still large numbers of women who think of the act of love as a "conjugal duty," enough to freeze anyone's pleasure in sex.

For problems of this kind, my own way of handling a consultation has proved quite successful. It has enabled me to help both men and women who find it difficult to talk about such things. When a man first enters my consulting-room, I can tell a great deal about him within a few seconds, just by looking at him. I notice whether he is fat and flabby or in good trim, and whether his movements are quick or slow, apathetic or aggressive, heavy or light. I pay particular attention to his eyes, for by their expression they reveal whether he is depressed, pessimistic, worried, cheerful, confident or mistrustful. Everything tells a tale. Even the shape of his face indicates to me his dominant characteristics, and by the condition of his skin, its hue and elasticity, I can judge whether he has a duodenal ulcer or liver trouble, whether he has high blood pressure, whether he is sexually maladjusted. The shape of his hands and the way he uses them tells me whether he's an intellectual or a workman. Also, certain details are very significant: if he bites his nails he isn't merely nervous or highly strung but a man with sexual problems. I have never known a virile, well-balanced man to bite his nails. His manner of dress is also a great give-away, and tells me at a glance whether the man is mean or stingy or cautious. Highly nervous and anxious men dress quite differently from calm and cheerful men.

My observations tell me even more about women. I know at a glance whether a woman is sexually frigid or fulfilled. The movements of a sensually happy and well-

adjusted woman are smooth and supple and somehow un-
hurried; she sways slightly from the hips, and her whole
body seems in tune. The movements of a frustrated woman
are much more jerky and mechanical, like a puppet, and
she is always highly strung. A frustrated woman is never
calm. Women also reveal a lot about themselves by the way
they dress. The frigid woman takes a lot of trouble over
her appearance, which is not surprising, since her energies
are all devoted to her clothes and make-up instead of being
channelled in other, more satisfying ways. She would like
to be seductive and exciting, and this is her way of com-
pensating for her lack of sexual satisfaction and deep fulfillment.

This is not the kind of thing you learn from books but by
experience. As soon as a patient enters the room, I know at
once whether or not I can be of help, and, by the same
token, whether or not I'll be able to cure him. I'm not the
only person to make these observations, of course. Every
good doctor works in this way, using his knowledge of
psychology and his intuition, and this explains why one
might be a highly qualified specialist and yet only a mediocre
doctor, or an obscure country doctor and yet a great practitioner.

I do not care for generalizations, especially in medicine,
and even less in sexual matters, where each case is so highly
individual. Nevertheless, one can divide these problems into
two major categories: organic and psychical. Organic problems are those that result from congenital or other malforma-
tions, and these, of course, are cases I cannot attempt to
cure. Psychical problems are the result of nervous or psychological disturbances, or are caused by such conditions as
infections or inflammation of the urinary system, diabetes,
albuminuria and especially obesity. For all these specific
conditions my plants are a powerful remedy.

When I am dealing with a sexual problem, my treatment
instructions always run to at least two pages, for in addition
to explaining how my basic prescription should be adminis-

tered I always prescribe a detailed diet: what the patient should eat and drink, and above all what he should avoid. Sometimes my prescriptions might not seem to have anything medical about them, but they are very effective. For example, for certain young women who are spinsters or are divorced and suffering from nervous depression due to frigidity or the lack of a man in their lives, I might prescribe: "Go alone on a trip to Italy," underlining *alone*. When the patient protests in alarm, "But that would be awful, I can't stand being alone as it is!" I tell her, "No, from the very first evening you must get out and about. Don't eat in the hotel restaurant, try the local specialties in little *trattorias*, take your coffee at a sidewalk café, go dancing—and believe me, you'll come back a different person."

It isn't that I think Italian men are any more gifted than others, but, especially in the south, they devote more time to their women. Their music and songs are sensual, and even the landscape is an enchantment. A woman is often cold because no one has ever devoted sufficient time or used the right means to arouse her. Women are, above all, sentimental creatures; they need pretty compliments to prepare them for the sexual act. An old-fashioned upbringing has often conditioned them to think of the act of love as something ugly, and if their first experience is a failure, and sometimes a painful failure, this only strengthens their erroneous ideas.

Men should always bear in mind the bowerbird. To welcome the female he prepares a sort of shelter on the ground which is to be their nuptial chamber. He tramples the soil with his little feet and removes anything that might hurt the delicate feet of his lady love, then he decorates the roof and walls of the house with flowers, and strews flowers over the ground. Only then does he fetch his wife, and amidst all the blazing colors, adorned like an Eastern prince, he puffs up his neck, lowers his head the better to display his aigrettes, and performs for her alone his love dance. What woman could resist such attentions and such beauty?

Very few couples enjoy a normal sex life. It sometimes takes very little to make a woman cold, for her sexual mechanism is very delicate. Contrary to what women too often think, man is not the coarse and brutish creature they imagine. The causes of impotence can be every bit as subtle as those that create problems in the sexual life of a woman. Nevertheless, I must positively state that, on my own findings, eighty-two out of a hundred women do not experience sexual fulfillment, and in 95 percent of these cases it is the man who is responsible.

The three problems I have most often encountered in men are: impotence, or desire with the physical ability to satisfy it; diminished sexual appetite, or lack of desire; premature ejaculation, or inability to achieve control. I dislike using these medical terms and never use them with my patients, because they seem to imply that the sexual act is a mechanical performance that can be expected to succeed every time. Such an idea gets in the way of the act of love, both as a thing of beauty and a satisfaction, and it certainly interferes with the cure of any difficulties that may have arisen.

It has been in matters of physical love that I have heard the saddest "confessions." There was, for example, the attractive and very lively young woman who confided to me:

"I am twenty-four and my husband is twenty-three, we've been married for six months and we still haven't had a wedding night. But I know he loves me. Before I met my husband I had a lover. I know the happiness a man can give me and I can't do without it any longer. I don't want to deceive my husband, so what can I do? I'm sleeping badly, I'm irritable, my nerves are on edge, I realize I'm getting impossible to live with. But when all night long I've felt the warmth of his body lying next to mine and my hand has felt the softness of his skin, then in the morning I just can't help it, I'm full of resentment. Yesterday, sir, I even called him impotent, and he wept like a child. I was shattered."

"Tell me, exactly what happens?"

"My husband kisses me for a long time; he likes that. I don't mind telling you that when we were engaged I used to think that if he did everything as well as he kissed, we were in for some fantastic times. The night we were married—he had his principles and he'd never touched me before—he kissed me and fondled me a bit and then he left me, saying, 'I can't help it, I love you so much, I've waited too long.' I believed him, but the next day and the next it was always the same."

"Perhaps you don't know that some men like to be courted a little by their wives?"

"Oh, no, sir, it takes two to make love, I know that. But he doesn't want me to touch him, it makes him angry."

"Has he ever told you why?"

"He just said, 'Leave that to the whores, it's bad enough that I'm not the first.' "

Now I understood. I gave her something to quiet her nerves and asked her to send her husband to see me.

"Every time we make love I can't help remembering that there was another man before me, and after that I just can't," he admitted.

"Do you love her?"

"I'm crazy about her."

I asked enough questions to learn that he had been given the strictest religious upbringing by his mother, a widow for many years, and that she had opposed his marriage. He even added: "And that was without knowing my wife had had a lover. If she'd known, she'd have forbidden me to marry her."

Finally, not being a highly sexed young man, he had never had a mistress, only a few brief encounters with prostitutes, which he said he had always regretted.

"But with them you weren't impotent?"

"No, it really wasn't possible."

His impotence was entirely in the mind. In his eyes, his relations with professional prostitutes had debased physical love to a vulgar act that he couldn't impose on the woman he loved, and his impotence was further aggravated by the thought that his wife had belonged to another. It took several conversations to rid him of his taboos, and my plants, by stimulating his desire, did the rest.

Other cases were not so easily treated. One day a pretty blonde woman, elegant and well-groomed, entered my consulting room. Mrs. W. came directly to the point, giving me the impression she had learned her confession by heart:

"When I was thirty-two it seemed as if all my dreams had come true. I married a man who was handsome and rich and kind, and in spite of the differences in our ages—he's fifty—I was sure I would be happy. My husband is a perfect man in every way, refined and attentive and very kind and above all not in the least self-centered, except when it comes to making love. Then I don't know him any more. He's abnormal. He hasn't made me happy even once, ever since we've been married!"

"Well now, had you ever enjoyed sex before you were married?"

"Of course. I had a lover and we got on perfectly."

"Did you by any chance get used to some kind of love-play that your husband perhaps dislikes or avoids?"

"I don't think so. Hans was very normal."

"I've no doubt of it, but butterflies spend a long time fluttering around the corolla before depositing their pollen into the heart of the flower, and perhaps these little pleasures were indispensable to you?"

She blushed so prettily that I felt sure her husband was to blame.

"Oh, no, sir."

I had asked her this question because it is frequently the case with women that they cannot do without the habits they formed when they were younger. It is a common problem with women of thirty to forty years old, particular in Anglo-Saxon countries, where they have practiced a lot of heavy petting with their boy friends. This might satisfy the demands of social hypocrisy, but it is sexually very trying and likely to cause serious inhibitions.

"No, sir, it really isn't my fault. You can't imagine how much I wish it were. With my husband it's the same thing every time. He comes into my bedroom, without warning, while I'm at my dressing-table. He comes close. I can tell he wants me, so I go and lie on the bed, and it's all over before he's even touched me. It sounds incredible, but I've never yet felt my husband inside me. The first time it happened I thought it was because his desire had been too fierce, but later I told him what a let-down it was for me. I could see that this made him wretched, and I was afraid it was a threat to our love, so I pretended to have an orgasm at the same time he did. This made him quite happy and he never seemed to grasp that it really wasn't possible. Then one day the whole pitiful farce made me scream with rage and anger. He thought I was screaming for joy, and ever since then I've screamed louder and louder. He doesn't realize that it's the animal scream of a body exhausted by this deception. It's driving me mad; I feel full of resentment towards him and I despise myself."

"Before anything else, I must see your husband."

She was right, he was handsome and charming and very manly. He told me that he had had his first orgasm when he was fifteen, in a dancer's dressing-room.

"She was sitting at her dressing-table and I stood behind her, watching. The dressing-room was filled with a heavy, erotic fragrance, the mingled odors of sweat and perfume and cosmetics, and I felt hot, but my hands were icy cold. She raised her arms and I saw the beads of sweat in her shaved armpits, and then I felt a sudden release. I thought I was going to faint, but afterwards I had a wonderful feeling of relief."

"Were you in love with this dancer?"

"I was mad about her, as boys are at that age."

"If you aren't in love with the woman, what happens?"

"I don't know. I've never made love to a woman I didn't love."

I talked with him about his sexual problems and treated his nervous system, and although it took a long time, the outcome was successful. Two years later Mrs. W. wrote to tell me she had given birth to a little girl, adding: ". . . and what's more, she isn't a test-tube baby!"

The way a couple behave when they come to see me is revealing. I allow the man and the woman a quarter of an hour each to explain their point of view, and then I wait. If the man speaks first, I know that I am dealing with an egoist and that there's little likelihood of his changing and becoming a considerate lover. I let him talk and then I turn to his wife. This kind of man generally interrupts her on every point, trying to make me think she has nothing of interest to add. I have noticed that such men are for the most part full-blooded fellows with necks like bulls, and they think themselves very virile because they are quickly aroused and quickly satisfied. It's their wives who come to me first, never they themselves, although Liliane S. and her husband were an exception.

In their case it was he who asked for the appointment. He was a man of about fifty, rather heavily built, with thick, short-cut, steely grey hair. His hands were on the stubby side, with broad palms, which indicates a fighter, the kind of man who gets into brawls of one kind or another. She was small and slender and seemed quite tiny next to him. There was an aura of good breeding about her; I noticed that she wore a touch of perfume and that her small and dainty feet were well shod. Her face was young, but her set lips betrayed a certain weariness and her expression was hard.

"My wife didn't want to come. She said it was pointless, since she's already asked for a divorce. And yet we've got a nice house, I've given her everything in the world that she wants: jewels, furs. She's got everything a woman could desire."

She straightened up in her chair and threw at him: "Everything except sex, Sir. My husband's impotent."

He reddened and the veins in his neck stood out.

"She's mad. We have five children, Sir." He turned to face her. "Did you get them by an impotent husband? That's feminine logic for you."

"Yes," she retorted, coolly ironical, "we have five children and you made them in fifty seconds."

One cannot say that the men of one country make love better than the men of another, but there are countries where men live at a less hectic pace. Men who live in cities, whatever their profession, are the most prone to sexual inadequacy because they live in a permanent state of tension, their nerves frayed by constant telephone calls and traffic jams and bills. In days gone by people lived more slowly and harmoniously. They had time to sit at the window and watch life go by, but nowadays this natural rhythm survives only in the country. The peasants in the Gers come to consult me about all sorts of ailments but rarely for problems of virility.

Whenever a man tells me that he has a cerebral approach to love-making, I know he's either impotent or afraid of becoming so. I recently had a very sad case of this very thing, which was destroying a happy marriage that had lasted over fifteen years. The wife was a delightful, pretty woman of about forty, with a peach-bloom complexion and soft dove-grey eyes. She was well dressed in a charming, slightly provincial way, and her voice was young, but with a bit of an edge to it.

"Sir, I can't stand my husband any longer. We've been sleeping in separate rooms for two years now, and I've hung on because I didn't want to admit that it was getting me down. I never thought much about whether my husband was handsome or whether he had a good physique—

good looks don't impress me—but my women friends used to envy me Lucien and say he was a good-looking man. All that counted to me was that I was happy in his arms. He used to call me his 'little bourgeoise,' because my love-making wasn't very sophisticated. I'd have loved to have had a child by him, but he wouldn't let me. He already had two children by a previous marriage and he didn't want them to suffer. At first we made love often, but as the years went by, less and less. I supposed it was only normal that we quieted down in this way, but then I found out that he had mistresses. I was dreadfully hurt, but when I told him he replied that he didn't have any feeling for them but that he needed certain kinds of excitement I wasn't able to provide.

"Of course, I was ready to try anything. He explained that while he still loved me as much as ever, there were more interesting ways of making love and that if you take your prejudices to bed with you they inhibit certain forms of sexual pleasure. For example if we were to be able to watch ourselves in a mirror when we were in each other's arms, it would be more subtly erotic and we'd get twice the enjoyment.

"Well, I accepted the mirrors without feeling too shocked, but then he became more demanding: he wanted me to meet other couples, to prove I loved him. We met in a hotel in Paris, and I thought we all seemed a bit ridiculous. They looked like depraved children with fifty-year-old wrinkles. It was a painful sight, and for me it quickly became horrible. I was watching my husband (who thinks he has a marvellous body) with another woman, and suddenly I saw that he had a paunch, a great fold of flesh across his stomach, hairy, spindly legs, and that his skin was all quivering. His body looked old and worn, older than his age. Blinded by love I had never noticed these things before.

"The whole thing was disgusting, and I decided that if this kind of sordid, indecent behavior was love, then I wanted to have no more to do with it. The next day I shut my bedroom door and made him sleep in the study. I've been very unhappy ever since, because I know that I'm missing something, and a couple who don't enjoy one another aren't a couple any more."

How right she was. There was really very little I could do for her. No amount of soothing baths can take the place of love. I saw her husband, and he was naturally unhappy that he'd lost his wife.

"But, sir," he said, "you must understand that I need these kinds of stimulation; without them I'd be impotent."

He was already halfway to being so.

"Why," I asked him, "did you make your wife participate in your experiments? You know the kind of person she is, you must have known she wouldn't be able to stand it."

"I loved her and I thought that with her it would be better than with the others."

In a way I pitied the man, but I felt angry with him too. He loved her, but not enough to give her a child, not enough to put their life together before his own pleasures. For people like him, my plants, my common sense and my knowledge of people are of no avail. I have not often had to admit defeat, but in the realm of sexual problems I have met more hopeless cases than in many other illnesses.

Mrs. Colette D. was thirty-eight, a bit on the plump side, exactly the kind of woman of whom men say: "I wouldn't mind taking her to bed!" The trouble was, she had lost interest. She was a nice, simple woman, not at all intellectual. She told me her trouble in simple terms:

"I'm afraid I can't help it, there's nothing I can do about it. As soon as my husband comes anywhere near me, I withdraw. I still love him, I love him a lot, but I can't bear having him touch me.

"It used to be good, making love with him. I'd really let myself go, you know how it is. I trusted him. He'd say: 'Don't worry about anything, I take precautions,' and I believed him. I was very young when I got married, only eighteen, and he was my first man, so I lacked experience.

And then one day I got caught. He said, 'We slipped up, don't worry, it won't happen again.' I believed him, but from eighteen to twenty-five I had five abortions. You see, we already had two children and we didn't want any more. My husband's very sensible about it. He says, 'It's one thing producing children, but it's another thing bringing them up.' Eventually, you know how women tell each other things, my friends said it was a bit much, that it was all his fault, all he had to do was . . . anyway, you know what I mean."

I knew one thing for certain, her husband was an egoist, a man with no will-power and no self-control.

". . . and I realized that what mattered to him was his own pleasure, and too bad about the consequences. But I was the one who paid for it, and so I learned to be careful. It was the same every time. When he started making love, I'd be quite happy, as long as there was no danger, but as soon as I felt myself getting carried away I'd go rigid with fear. To keep from letting myself go I only had to think of the frantic worry when my next period was due. I'd visualize all the humiliating performance I'd have to go through and all the pain I'd have to put up with, and I'd push him away and let him have his climax by himself. I don't even have to think about it any more, it's automatic. I push him away and I'm left feeling frustrated, my nerves on edge. He doesn't want me to take the pill either, but anyway I think it's too late to make any difference. As far as I can see, sex is just a rotten business that works only for men. Now, when he makes love to me, I don't feel anything at all. I've become frigid."

Frigidity from fear of pregnancy is very common. The woman often pushes the man away before the climax and, cheated of her orgasm, she gradually becomes physically unresponsive. Sometimes to avoid this frustration, a woman quickly learns the safe way to achieve orgasm, but this soon becomes a sexual habit necessary to her enjoyment, and thereafter ordinary love-making leaves her cold.

Some of the most extraordinary reactions one encounters

are among very young women. One, for example, assured me that she was completely and irrevocably frigid, telling me that she had only enjoyed sex with another woman. "But," she said, "I know it couldn't have been a real orgasm because it wasn't a man who was giving it to me." She preferred to think of herself as frigid rather than admit to any sexual abnormality.

Another young woman explained:

"I was very tempted to take a man of forty as a lover. Several of my friends had been telling me that boys of our own age are no good at making love. I knew an older man might know more ways of making me happy than a husband my own age, but on the other hand I didn't see why you should necessarily be clumsy just because you're young. Besides, with a young husband we'd be learning together, and what we didn't know wouldn't matter. I wouldn't miss it if I'd never known it anyway."

I don't pretend to give courses on sexual education. What advice I give is merely to help those who come to me to live sexually fulfilled and happy lives. My methods are simple. First and foremost I ban any of the aphrodisiacs that are sold under the counter, for these one-night stimulants are highly dangerous and can even cause heart attacks, and, if they are taken in excess, they can actually have the reverse effect and make a man completely impotent.

My treatment consists of foot-baths and vaginal douches, along with regular massage at the base of the spine with a highly effective cream made from plants. Patients have telephoned me to say that they have been amazed at the results, even after using the cream for only a short time, and some women have assured me that they felt the effects of these massages almost immediately. The cream is made from three plants: greater celandine, cow-parsnip and summer savory, and in certain cases I also add peppermint and broad-leaved plantain.

The celandine should be fresh, not more than fifteen to eighteen days old. This is why I never treat impotence dur-

ing the months of January and February, but in March the
sap is flowing and rising again and giving the plants amazing new strength, which they in their turn pass on. Spring
is the best time for treating sexual deficiencies.

Cow-parsnip, which my father used to call "Bear's Paw,"
is recommended by Dr. H. Leclerc [1] as a natural aphrodisiac
without side effects. His experiments with cases of genetic
debility were most conclusive.

Savory, according to one legend, is supposed to have been
named, aptly, after the satyrs, those jolly horned and hairy
creatures, half man and half billy-goat, who were forever
playing pipes and dancing and making love to gentle
nymphs, and who were so well endowed by nature that
they could turn a great many maidens into grown women
in the course of a single day. The origin of the name is perhaps debatable, but the results obtained with this plant are
not. Dr. J. Valnet [2] also recognizes it as a remarkable stimulant, both to the body and the mind.

To help my "miracle plants" do their work, I advise a
certain physical regimen and an effective diet. It is a mistake to make love too often, for human stamina is not inex-
haustible, and it is a medically attested fact that sexual
overactivity is one of the possible causes of impotence. By
the same token, any excessive physical exertion that calls
on man's reserves of nerve and muscle can, during periods
of intensive training, for example, result in temporary impotence and possible serious aftereffects.

I highly recommend walking, in forests or in the country
or by the sea (iodine is an excellent stimulant). Walking
has a relaxing and calming effect, without taking away the
desire for certain other pleasant forms of physical exercise.
Spirits should be avoided, and wine drunk only in moderation. All alcoholics are impotent, and a man who is really
drunk is unable to finish what he has started. An excess

[1] A leading authority on phytotherapy.
[2] *Aromathérapie*. Paris, Maloine, 1964.

of tobacco or any other stimulant that upsets the nervous system is similarly inadvisable.

As for the ravages caused by those chemical pep pills, which are designed to keep you awake when your whole system is crying out for sleep, what can one say? And what about the "happy pills," which are designed to make you forget your worries and cares and override your physical and mental exhaustion, thus turning you into a perfect candidate for nervous depression and impotence? After you've wakened up you have to get to sleep, so you soon start taking sleeping-pills, in increasing amounts. With the help of these three destructive agents, your day becomes very short, however late you stay up, and you no longer have time to make love. Besides, you soon stop even thinking about it, and when you do think of it, not perhaps from any real desire but because you are close to a woman you actually love, you no longer have the ability.

Cut out all stimulants and, instead, eat plenty of salt-water fish, brains, and shellfish, all rich in phosphorus, the phosphorus you are expending each day in physical, mental and sexual activity.

Also, take moderate amounts of certain spices: pepper, cinnamon, nutmeg, paprika. Eat plenty of celery too. There's certainly some truth in the popular belief that celery makes a person amorous.

19

A Fascinating Monster: Farouk

A surfeit of sex can also lead to loss of sexual appetite. If every dish you eat is highly spiced, by the end of the meal your mouth is so fiery you can't taste a thing. If every day you were fed only the most choice and delicate dishes, you'd long for a good peasant meal of boiled fowl.

King Farouk was the most spoiled, indulged man in the world. He didn't need to lift a finger to have his every desire and whim gratified. He wasn't a big man; he was just a fat man whose aggressiveness was aggravated by his obesity.

When I met Farouk, I was still giving consultations at the Majestic in Nice. That afternoon I had just had a tiring drive from Lyon, and my secretary greeted me with: "Sir, King Farouk wants to see you. He's already called twice."

This flattering news naturally tickled my vanity, and I kept wondering who could have told him about me. I was examining a lady who had a stall in the fish market when my secretary opened the door—a thing she normally would never do—and said, "Sir, it's the King on the telephone again!"

The lady from the fish market was unable to contain herself: "Don't keep him waiting! Just think of that now, a king. What a bit of luck I came today. I'll wait outside. You can call me back when you've finished."

The man on the phone spoke with an Italian accent, and I subsequently learned that his name was Gino and that he was the King's right-hand man.

"His Majesty King Farouk wishes you to come and see him."

I've never been very hot on the niceties of protocol, and I must also admit that I hadn't at that time had much experience of such things.

"I'm greatly honored," I replied, and added, "what day and what time?"

"His Majesty would like you to come at once."

It was on the tip of my tongue to say, "I'm with a patient," but then, after all, it was King Farouk who wanted to see me.

"Where?"

"In Monte Carlo, where His Highness is staying. We have booked rooms for you in the Hotel de Paris. His Majesty will see to it that you have everything you want."

I replied in a voice I hoped sounded blasé. "That will be quite all right."

"May we be allowed to send the Rolls for you immediately?"

"I have my own car."

"His Majesty would like you to use the Rolls; he thinks it will be nicer for you."

This brought out the peasant-revolutionary in me, crying "Down with the tyrants!" My car was as good as a king's and I'd go in it if I wanted to.

"I have my own car and a chauffeur, and anyway I enjoy driving."

I didn't have a chauffeur, of course, but this apparently made an impression on the secretary because he didn't press the point, and I opened my door again to call back the lady from the fish market.

"I say, was he a real king then; it's not someone pulling your leg?"

At seven o'clock I drew up outside the Hotel de Paris. The

bellboys, the porter with all his gold braid, and a dark young man wearing a fez were milling round me almost before I'd opened the car door. The country boy in me thought: Heavens, I wonder how much all this costs in tips, but the man-of-the-world Mességué said, "Will you show me to my rooms?"

The hall-porter leaped forward, only to be stopped by the young man who turned out to be His Majesty's third secretary.

"No, no," he said, "Mr. Mességué is expected. I'll take him to his rooms myself."

We walked through two of my rooms into a third, which was full of flowers, where His Majesty's first secretary was waiting. He took my briefcase, which was empty—I'd brought it only to make a good impression—and another rather thick-set man greeted me.

"It was I who telephoned."

There was a short silence, and I expected him to take me to the King. Instead he opened the door into the next room.

"This is your bedroom, you may have a rest."

"But I'm not tired. I'd rather you took me straight to the King."

"His Majesty is very busy, you might have a long wait. Order anything you wish, but don't leave your rooms. I will come and fetch you when His Majesty is ready to see you."

I was left by myself, feeling foolish; an army expression, "hurry up and wait" came to mind, as I stood there in the middle of my huge bedroom. I hadn't envisaged being kept waiting like a prisoner, but the "cell" was beautiful and comfortable. It was an amazing room: there was a very wide, low bed covered in black satin, beige carpets as thick and springy as an English lawn, occasional tables, pink and green opalines and two pale-blue telephones. The bathroom, which was big enough for a dining-room for a large family, was all in marble and black-and-gold mosaics, and the inside of the vast bathtub was a subtle shade of turquoise blue. The fabulous view from my window was like a picture postcard: the violet sea, the white rock of the Principality, and the white-and-red flag of Monaco, which seemed shot with gold as it fluttered above the palace in the light of the setting sun.

It was irritating to find myself at the beck and call of this invisible Majesty, but it had been a tiring day so I loosened my tie, stretched out on the bed and shut my eyes.

I was awakened by the discreet tinkle of the telephone.

"His Majesty will receive you in a few minutes. I'll come and fetch you."

According to my watch it was 4:30 in the morning. I put on my jacket, mechanically feeling in the pockets as one usually does, and discovered that I'd forgotten my pendulum. Clearly, at that hour in the morning it would be impossible to get hold of one anywhere in Monaco, but I noticed that there were heavy brass knobs dangling from the curtain cord. I cut the cord and removed a knob, and after that all I needed was to ask the chambermaid for a bit of cotton, and I had a perfect pendulum. Luckily I've never considered my pendulum a magic instrument, and the thought of examining His Majesty with a brass knob from a curtain cord actually had its funny side.

Gino was back in ten minutes. "Follow me, please."

Corridors, elevator, more corridors, another elevator. I began to wonder if I was still dreaming.

"Where are we going?"

"This elevator goes to the underground passage."

"What underground passage?"

"That leads to His Majesty's rooms."

Now I was sure I was dreaming. No consultation had ever led me to such strange circumstances.

"His Majesty is gambling in his private rooms at the Casino," Gino explained, "and this underground passage leads there directly from the Hotel de Paris."

A few moments later we were entering a cream-and-gold

salon. There, seated at a gambling-table, wearing a loose-fitting raw-silk suit, his enormous neck emerging from a shirt with narrow pink stripes, sat His Majesty King Farouk. He was finishing his twenty-seventh game that night, or so I was told, and close at hand I observed two bottles of champagne on ice, a huge open jar of caviar and a mountain of cold chicken legs.

The table was covered in green baize and illuminated by a harsh light that cast deep shadows on the hands and faces of the players. An expressionless croupier held the bank, and around Farouk were four other men and two women of about fifty. There was no doubt that they were addicts, the kind of people for whom gambling is a substitute for sex. Their bed of pleasure was the table, their thrill was losing, their satisfaction was winning. They got their sensual kicks, reflected in their hollowed cheeks and trembling hands, from the fascinating movement of those chips, as the croupier raked them in or pushed them towards them, and from the cards they grasped as they came out of the polished mahogany shoe. When the night was over they would be drained—mentally, physically and sometimes financially.

I looked at "my patient." From his photographs I had expected a man with black hair and brown eyes, but I saw that what hair he still had was light chestnut. He had just noticed me and was looking at me strangely, with cold blue eyes. He struck me as very intelligent. His face was smooth and unlined and showed no signs of fatigue. In contrast with the exhausted players around him, he seemed extraordinarily lively. Yet I was uneasy in his presence, for I felt there was something unnatural about him. He smiled at me, showing his very white carnassial teeth, and instantly I understood the kind of seductive fascination this obese tyrant could still have. Politely he asked: "Ah, Mr. Mességué, do you mind waiting while I finish this hand?"

I wasn't expected to reply, of course. He gambled royally. One evening his opponent had pointed out to him that he had shown only three kings of the carré or four-of-a-kind, that he had called. He had replied: "And with me, the King of Egypt, doesn't that make four?"

What I had heard of him as a man was that he gobbled up a dozen eggs for breakfast, ate two-pound steaks, and that once in a restaurant in Rome he had ordered twenty cutlets and then, having eaten only nineteen of them, had left the twentieth for the *maître d'hôtel*, saying: "Here you are, a share for the poor!"

This, then, was the man I was observing. I was no longer uneasy or timid, and I knew that soon I would be examining him. He would be in my hands and, just like the woman from the fish market, he'd be looking into my eyes for the promise that he could be cured. There certainly wasn't anything seriously wrong with him. He radiated an extraordinary life force, but he would have to be put on a diet and I foresaw that this would not be easy.

"Come over here, Mr. Mességué."

Calmly he threw a half-eaten drumstick over his shoulder and wiped his hand on his trousers. At a sign from him the waiter offered me a glass of champagne, which I refused.

"Would you prefer a Scotch?"

I said no to that too, as well as to the chicken legs and pastries and the Havana cigar His Majesty had offered me. I saw a flicker of angry surprise in his eyes.

"You are very hard to please, Mr. Mességué. And this?"

He snapped his fingers and a blonde young woman came up to me. She brushed against me, apparently ready to gratify my every desire. I was spared any answer, for Farouk continued: "Anyway, that'll keep until later." He gave a quite nasty laugh. "Now you can watch a man lose to order, because I'm the King. This gentleman is my minister, he does what I tell him."

He indicated a man of about fifty, rather thick-set, as dark-skinned as myself, with dark, heavy eyelids, who was endeavoring to maintain an impassive expression. Discreetly, the other players withdrew.

From the other side of the table the minister shot me a quick look, and the expression in his eyes, the glimmer of panic, put me in mind of a hunted animal. Gino whispered to me, "Above all, keep quiet."

"Deal the cards," Farouk commanded.

The croupier gave out the cards.

"Lose," ordered Farouk, "and don't cheat."

I could see the beads of perspiration on the minister's forehead, like one of those screen close-ups. Farouk put down his cards. They were good, and the minister looked relieved. Then he put down his own, which, fortunately, were less good.

"He doesn't even need to cheat, he loses to order. What do you call that in France? Filth . . . that's what he is, that's what they all are."

He repeated the coarse term with apparent enjoyment; by now all I wanted was to go home. But with a gesture he summoned back his harem, sat the blonde on his knees and started stroking her hips with his enormous ring-laden hand.

"She's got nothing under her dress, not even her conscience —she hasn't got one."

Then he sent them all away. The show was over.

"Now, Mr. Mességué, we'll talk about me. I'll tell you why I asked you to come."

This was the first time I'd ever given a consultation in a casino gambling-room, but I examined Farouk with my pendulum as conscientiously as I'd have done in my own consulting-room. Then I made out my prescription for hand- and foot-baths. I never reveal my patients' ailments unless they are already public knowledge, such as Herriot's rheumatism or Churchill's cough, so I won't say what plants I used for His Majesty. They gave good results, however, since he subsequently asked me to see him at Koubbah, near Cairo.

His palace was extraordinary, but cold. There wasn't a single room, a single corner, where you felt that the furnishings had been placed by a loving hand. It was like a dream from the Thousand and One Nights that bordered on nightmare.

About a year had passed since I'd seen Farouk in Monte Carlo, and I found him greatly altered. He had lost practically all his hair and was considerably fatter. His eyes were sunk in unpleasant layers of fat, and a glint of cruel scorn now gleamed permanently between his lazily drooping eyelids.

He held out his hand and greeted me with surprising warmth: "Welcome to my home." He was surrounded by his ministers, his dignitaries bedecked in all their finery, his courtiers, his secretaries.

His servants, muscular giants or listless young men with magnificent Oriental eyes, plied to and fro, silent and attentive.

"Gentlemen, let me introduce Mr. Mességué. I command you to be treated by him and to see to it that he has a very pleasant time here. You may leave us. Mességué, come with me, I'll show you a few knick-knacks."

He had a priceless collection of music-boxes, of which he was very proud.

"Look at them, they've got as much life in them as my ministers—always doing the same things, going through the same set of motions."

His antique watches, several hundred of them, were real works of art, in gold and precious stones and enamels, and were even then worth hundreds of millions.

Gino was respectfully following us, and he whispered: "It's a great honor to be shown round by the King." Personally, I could have happily done without Farouk while I looked at all these marvellous things, for his comments were very grating:

"I get a kick out of owning these things that other men once thought were theirs forever. It didn't take much money to make them mine. Here's General Kléber's toilet-case. There's the Czar's thermometer; it's set with gold and diamonds, as if the place where he stuck it stank less than other men's! The baton with the golden eagle and the red iron cross was a gift from Hitler to Marshal von Brauchi'tsch. And the snuff-box belonged to Frederick the Great. What I like is the inscription: 'I belonged to Frederick I. Frederick II gave me to his son and I must be kept in the family.' Amusing, don't you think?"

On the wall of his study hung the portrait of a very handsome, slim young man with a gentle, almost childlike expression: King Farouk when he was sixteen.

"Yes, yes, that's me. You're thinking I don't look like that now. It was painted in 1936 when I came to the throne. I've altered, haven't I?"

He was unrecognizable, yet he was only thirty, this obese, bald-headed colossus of a man. He indicated a clenched fist in bronze on the huge inlaid table that served as his desk.

"You've doubtless heard of this? Yes, Mességué, whatever I want, that's how I get it."

I was finding him even more loathsome than at Monte Carlo and thinking that at this rate the monarchy in Egypt couldn't last much longer.

"Mr. Mességué, you read men's bodies, I read their minds. I'm clairvoyant too. I know quite well that there are only five kings in the world who'll survive: the king of hearts, the king of clubs, the king of diamonds, the king of spades—and the King of England.

"A man can have a very pleasant time when he visits Koubbah. Make the most of it while you're here; our Oriental nights are very beautiful."

That evening, in my fairy-tale bedroom with its silks and gold and Oriental rugs and soft lights and perfumes and music drifting in, I found twin sisters waiting for me. They were very lovely, with doe eyes and perfect bodies, and their every movement, their dances, their very voices, held a sensuous, heady fascination. For them, love was a ritual; they performed each gesture with a kind of religious fervor.

They were the priestesses the Egypt of the Pharaohs had known.

My bed was huge and covered with cushions, and stood on a dais. Farther on in my suite of rooms was a pink marble pool, filled with water that was strangely blue and soft, and after each embrace the sisters would go and bathe, and pour perfume over each other. It was an intoxicating performance. Then they would bring me fruit and honey cakes stuffed with nuts, pistachios and almonds and treacherous spices, and rose quince with hashish. Towards the middle of the night two naked black women came on the scene, their bodies smooth and perfectly formed, and massaged the two sisters with fragrant oils. Then they turned to me, and under their skillful hands my fatigue melted away and I felt supple and fresh and as good as new. Two black men served me a sweet wine the color of pale amber that tasted of cinnamon. It was all marvellously well-orchestrated, and I'd never have believed it could exist outside of novels or Hollywood spectaculars, but for me, for one night, it was real.

To arouse my appetite or quench my returning thirst, the two velvet-eyed gazelles were ready to do anything I might ask of them. Sadist? I only had to raise my hand. At a signal from me, the black women were ready to crack the whips that hung from their belts. Masochist? They were at my disposal. Everything had been thought of. I had only to ask and any tableau of the Oriental nights would come to life. My tastes were more modest and I was quite content with the twin sisters, but I must admit that I made the most of that unusual night, nor would I believe any normal man who claimed he had resisted such an assault upon his senses.

When I woke up next morning, the sun had long since risen over Egypt. It could all have been a dream: I was alone, not a thing in the room was out of place, the fountain in the pool was scattering diamonds in the sunshine, silence reigned. I lay there thinking things over and I began to see how if a man had all this, nights like this whenever he fancied, he'd soon start needing something else. And before long he'd become another King Farouk. Silently I thanked my father for making me what I am, and I thanked God for never letting me forget him.

Twenty-four hours later I left the palace, and from the plane I could see the tiny black figures of the fellahs, like insects, scratching away at the age-old land of the Pharaohs. That was the last time I saw Farouk. He never asked me again to Egypt, and I was glad of it, for I cannot be sure I'd have had the courage to resist the sweet and gentle gazelles of the palace of Koubbah.

20

Utrillo's Hands and Cocteau's Heart

I DON'T CARE MUCH for statistics. It's a modern craze that I don't share, and I'm particularly uneasy about the use of statistics in relation to illness. To transform sick people into facts and figures is to make them part of the country's economy, much like meat prices or petroleum output.

It would never have entered my mind to convert the results of my own treatments into statistics, but one of my colleagues did so for me. He spent countless evenings going through all my patients' cards, which we then listed in three categories: (1) cured; (2) improvement; (3) recurrence, failure or unknown, the last meaning that the patient failed to return and never let us know the results of his treatment.

This is the first time I have ever derived such pleasure from a list of figures:

	CURED	IMPROVEMENT	RECURRENCE, FAILURE OR UNKNOWN
Angina pectoris and infarction	50%	40%	10%
Arteritis	15	70	15
Arthritis	30	60	10

	CURED	IMPROVEMENT	RECURRENCE, FAILURE OR UNKNOWN
Asthma	60	30	10
Chronic bronchitis	10	80	10
Chronic rheumatism	30	65	5
Circulatory disorders	80	10	10
Colon bacillus infection	60	30	10
Disturbances of the sympathetic nervous system	85	10	5
Ears, nose and throat	40	30	30
Eczema	98		2
Emphysema	10	70	20
Hemorrhoids	50%	20%	30%
Heart	50	40	10
Insomnia	80	10	10
Intestinal complaints	50	30	20
Migraines	80	10	10
Edema	30	60	10
Prostate	50	40	10
Sciatica	60	30	10
Stomach	80	15	5
Tension	30	30	40
Urea	50	30	20
Varicose ulcers	30	30	40

Yet these statistics, flatteringly eloquent though they are, don't really convey very much to me, whereas a name, suddenly remembered, will recall the battle we fought, the patient and I, against his illness. I cannot do without the patient's cooperation any more than a doctor can; the patient's faith is indispensable to his cure. Sometimes the name of a complaint will summon memories to my mind. If I think of asthma, for example, I recall very vividly the amazing episode of Narcose Murciano in Morocco.

I had been invited to deliver four lectures in Casablanca, to be followed by a question period. The audience was animated, as always in those lands of sunshine, and many people had already attended the previous lectures, following them like episodes of a serial. I owed my success in part to four doctors who had turned up each evening to "represent the opposition" and uphold traditional medicine. In those days I still tended to identify the Medical Council, which was taking me to court again and again, with doctors themselves, and I had often leaped swiftly to the attack in my own defense. Our polite but impassioned arguments appealed to the public, and outside the lecture hall the sidewalk cafés and squares were always full of pro- and anti-Mességués loudly and animatedly arguing the toss.

At question time that evening, things became heated. One of the doctors—Dr. Corcos I think it was—stood up and said: "Mr. Mességué, I don't doubt your honesty and your good faith, I merely doubt the efficacy of your treatments. Like St. Thomas, I believe only what I see for myself."

I was carried away by my natural ardor, and replied:

"Let me make you a proposition: you choose a patient, I'll take him back on the plane with me, I'll treat him, I'll keep him for two or three months, I'll pay all his expenses and give him whatever salary he'd have been earning in Morocco. My only condition is this—that he be examined by the same panel of doctors at his departure and on his return."

"I accept, sir, on condition that we choose the patient."

"That's all right, only I ask the right to choose the illness."

"Choose."

"Asthma."

The audience was delirious, everyone shouting and jumping up and down. This was the second time I'd made such a proposition in North Africa in the course of a lecture. The African sun must have gone to my head for me to indulge in such folly! I could hear my father's voice: "If you stick your finger in the fire, my son, you can expect to get burned."

The hall had barely calmed down when a gentleman got to his feet: Max Hymans, Director General of Air France.

"Sir, Air France will be happy to offer the patient a return ticket."

I was to meet my patient the following day. He was a hairdresser, Narcose Murciano, father of five children, who was suffering from such severe chronic asthma that work had become impossible. His acute attacks were so serious that the last one had very nearly killed him. His case was desperate.

When I saw him, I thought, I'm done for. This man isn't just ill, he's dying. He'll die on my hands. I've the right to refuse him. I'm no more a miracle-worker than a doctor is. I'll ask them to give me another patient. While these thoughts were milling round in my head, I was examining him. His skin had lost all its elasticity—it stuck together when you pinched it, like a sick dog's. The four opposition doctors were all present, and one of them very decently called me aside: "We hadn't seen him recently; we didn't realize he was in such a bad way, so you needn't be ashamed of refusing."

I was on the point of doing so when my patient, between gasps, managed to say: "Sir, take me with you, you're my last hope. My children need me."

His magnificent black eyes held my own. I have never forgotten those eyes, which expressed all the anguish of a man who feels the hand of death upon his shoulder. I accepted.

The journey to France was a nightmare. The poor wretch had to be so careful not to waste any of what life he still had left that he made not the slightest movement. He even kept his eyes shut. In the face of such a desperate will to live, I gained new heart. I wasn't going to fight alone, this man would be helping me.

Two months later I took him back to Casa, completely cured, and he has had no more attacks to this day. For me, I admit, this was a fine victory, and since then the doctors in Morocco have sent me every asthmatic who has failed to respond to traditional treatment.

My highest percentage of cures—98 percent—has been

with eczema; it was this that brought about my introduction to Maurice Utrillo.

At that time I still sometimes gave people appointments myself. That I no longer do so is not conceit but caution, for I would regularly forget to tell my secretary what appointments I had made, with the result that sometimes two or three people would turn up at the same time. On this particular day my secretary had booked a Lucie Valore for 4:30, but as I had made one of my triple appointments, I had to keep Lucie Valore and her husband waiting for two hours. I had no idea who she was, this opulent-looking woman covered in necklaces, pearls and gold bracelets and swathed in the kind of shawls that hippies would rave about today. Waiting with her was a wizened, nervous, jumpy old man, whom I blithely assumed to be Mr. Valore, his navy blue suit hanging loosely on his emaciated body. Soon afterwards I learned that this old man was Maurice Utrillo.

Lucie Valore made a memorable entrance into my consulting-room, sailing majestically in like a great galleon laden with Aztec spoils.

"You may sit down," she told me, "and you, too, Maurice, and be sure you do everything the gentleman says. It's about him that I've come, Sir. I'll tell you what's wrong with him. He drinks too much and it's giving him eczema. Show the gentleman your leg, Maurice, and your hands."

Docilely he held out his hands, which trembled like two panic-stricken old birds. They were hands of astonishing beauty in their old age, with the spatula-shaped thumbs that might have belonged to a sculptor.

"We're two great painters, you know," she went on. "Unfortunately, Maurice has great difficulty in painting and even in signing his name, which is really very annoying, as his signature's worth a lot of money. What can you do for him?"

"Before I answer that, I'll have to examine him and ask him a few questions."

"Then it would be better if you came to Le Vésinet. Maurice doesn't feel well here, the place lacks beauty. Maurice is used to being surrounded by my works of art, he can't live without them. You'll see our paintings for yourself when you come. It'll make your consultation more interesting."

I accepted without hesitation, for I was anxious to see this couple against their own background. As I pushed open the gate of their villa, in the Rue Cortot in Le Vésinet, I thought nothing could surprise me. I was wrong. To me, with my love of unspoiled nature, the garden looked dreadfully small. The grounds were dotted with little rococo statues, and the complicated twists and turns of the garden paths put me in mind of a miniature golf course. At the end of the garden stood a house[1] of no specific style, with rough-cast faded pink walls and attics. At the entrance to the garden stood a chapel, which in size and architecture made one think of the chapels you find in cemeteries.

The house was more like a museum. As I entered I glimpsed on the right the "Salle Valadon," which served as a drawing-room, its walls hung with twenty-three paintings by Maurice Utrillo's mother. I was later to have the opportunity of admiring these masterpieces. On the left was the "Salle Utrillo." I couldn't say what color the walls were, for they were covered from floor to ceiling by the master's canvases, but I had time to read a card in Utrillo's handwriting: "In creating Lucie, God created my happiness."

The main room, which served as a living-room, was devoted to "Utrillo-Valore." There were plenty of Valores but very few Utrillos. This was where I was received by Lucie, enthroned in an easy-chair, the diamonds glittering on her plump hands as she stroked one of her favorite Pekinese, a snuffly, smelly little dog, while the other four yapped jealously at her feet.

"I must introduce you to my darlings: Choudi, Chou-

[1] Now the Utrillo Museum.

Chou, Utrillette, Valorette, Marquise. They don't like strangers."

One could barely make oneself heard, for there was also a large aviary in the room, containing about thirty parakeets, all making a deafening racket. Standing silent in a corner, chewing on a cigarette butt, ashes all over his suit, Utrillo was looking at me. His eyes were a washed-out, forget-me-not blue, full of poignant sadness.

Under the watchful and imperious eye of the woman whom Maurice, on his submissive days, would call *"Ma bonne Lucie,"* I examined this great painter, who had the air of an abandoned child. As I questioned him I kept seeing another face between us: the face of Schoum, the tramp. Maurice Utrillo's eczema had a similar cause—red wine—so I decided to use approximately the same preparations. However, as the painter's nerves were in a much worse state than Schoum's had been, I also added buttercup, sweet briar and peppermint. There could be no question of putting him on a diet, so I merely prescribed hand- and foot-baths, and he did, in fact, follow this treatment for some time, with good results.

The consultation finished, Lucie embarked on initiating me into her painting.

"Have a good look at this canvas, now. It's a portrait I did of Rita Hayworth. Prince Ali Khan had commissioned Maurice to do it—it was to be his wedding present to Rita —but naturally Maurice refused. He told them: 'I can paint a house or a street for you, but not your wife. I never paint women, except for *ma bonne Lucie.*' So to help them out I did this portrait, and then they said they weren't interested. I was especially annoyed, as I'd had a lot of trouble with it. I can only paint real beauty, the beauty of the mind and soul, and she had absolutely none. She didn't have a face, she had a mask painted by Hollywood."

I found Lucie's paintings very ugly: a lot of loud, vulgar colors applied so thickly that I felt like asking her if she painted with a trowel. Utrillo meanwhile was getting bored. He sat down at a harmonium and started playing, but childishly, producing a series of droning, nasal sounds. Through the yapping of the dogs and the chattering of the parakeets, I could hear his quavering voice singing a hymn.

"He's very religious, you know. He's a great mystic. Maurice, introduce Mr. Mességué to your friends on your harmonium."

Next to a plaster statuette of St. Paul were photographs of Sacha Guitry and Maurice Chevalier, the latter inscribed: "From one Maurice to another."

Regal as ever, Lucie dismissed me with: "I shan't see you out. If you want to see a few paintings before you leave, you may have a look round."

There was something heart-rending about Maurice Utrillo's mysticism. Several times when I arrived at the villa I found him kneeling on the ground in his chapel, sunk in prayer at the foot of a frightful statue of the Sacred Heart of Mary, while the rosary he held in his trembling hands would rattle against the stone slabs of the floor. It required the Good Lord at his very gates to calm this tormented spirit. There was a story behind this little chapel. Maurice had begged Lucie to have it built for him, and then he had wanted it to be consecrated. Accordingly, one Sunday morning the curé of Le Pecq had come, in his surplice, with two choir boys, and since then Maurice seemed to have recovered a degree of composure. But goodness knows how "good" and "obedient" he must have been to obtain all that, Lucie had made him paint a certain number of pictures for it.

I have never witnessed such painful scenes as I did in that house. There were constant ugly rows between Lucie and him, and he would answer in the same gutter vocabulary as her own, their mildest insults being "cretin" and "slut." I heard more foul language in my few visits to the villa than I'd heard in fifteen years from all my patients put together, Farouk included.

Maurice, who had never been cured of his "addiction," in spite of numerous cures and spells of confinement, would start shouting: "Give me some wine, you slut!"

At times like this she was no longer his *"bonne Lucie."*

"Go and get—"

"Bitch, bitch, bitch . . ."

"I'll give you some if you'll tell Mr. Mességué I'm a greater painter than your mother."

"You'll give me some wine? A whole bottle? Without water?"

"Yes. After all, Mességué, you've only got to look at this canvas" (showing me her latest work) "to see it's worth more than any Valadon. It has the freedom of genius, it takes flight, whereas that poor Suzanne with her thick, heavy brush-strokes was floundering. Admit it, Maurice. You don't want to say it just because she was your mother. He was crazy about her, the cretin . . ."

"My wine!"

"You'll get it, but first say it."

"No, first give me the bottle."

"Look, here it is."

She showed him the bottle, and with shining eyes and trembling lips, Maurice held out his hands for it, jabbering: "You're gifted, Lucie, you're very gifted."

"Say it, say: 'More than my mother.' "

"Go to blazes with your bottle."

And the poor man began to cry, yet I think he was happy because he hadn't betrayed his mother.

When Lucie had exhausted this topic she would start on another: "Maurice, Pétrides [1] wants a 'snow,' dear. Do him a snow. It's what you do best and it's worth millions. Do it for him."

"No. I'll do him a spring, but I'm sick of doing snows. I want to slap some green and pink on a canvas. White gives me the shivers."

These scenes generally took place upstairs in Maurice's

[1] Paul Pétrides, Utrillo's dealer.

studio, which smelled of smoke and stale tobacco. Maurice used to spit out his fag ends all over the place.

"Do a snow and I'll double your wine ration?"

"Two bottles?"

And so, defeated, he would start on a new canvas, squeezing his tubes of paint lavishly on to his palette. Maurice Utrillo was copying himself. He no longer had anything new to say. I don't pretend to know much about painting, but I could see the difference between what he was producing now and the pictures that hung in the "Salle Utrillo," the finest of which dated back to 1912.

Eventually I managed to tame my patient, and looking at me with those pathetic eyes of his, he would say: "You know, dear boy, I'm very fond of you, but why do you have to soak your herbs in water? I don't like water."

"It makes no difference since you don't drink it."

And he would laugh like a broken puppet. Sometimes, when Lucie left us alone for a few moments, he would point to himself:

"Look at me. Look what she's done to me. She's turned me into a bourgeois. That's why I drink, I have to forget."

He had a lot to forget: his childhood, his poverty, the death of his mother. The more Utrillo came to trust me, the more Lucie grew suspicious, and my biggest mistake was when, clumsily, I criticized her latest "work of art."

"Tell me frankly what you think of it, Mességué. Don't worry, I won't take any notice of what you say, *I* know what it's worth."

It was worth a lot, since she forced anyone who bought a Utrillo to take a Lucie Valore too. What's more, she didn't give it away, she always charged a high price. I kept quiet.

"Come on, you must have *some* opinion?"

Yes, an opinion best not expressed.

"What do you see in the painting?"

"Ears of corn."

"You can see a face, can't you? Do you recognize who it is?"

"No."

"It's Danièle Delorme. I've captured her very soul, and there it is, like a butterfly nailed to a wall."

She was getting on my nerves, and I was disgusted with the way she kept tormenting Utrillo, so finally I let myself go: "Perhaps it's what you say. But you're the only one to see it. To normal people, like me, it's just a pile of paint."

I thought she was going to beat me up. You could see the anger rising in her like a great wave; it was almost beautiful.

"You're a nincompoop, a dull-witted, ignorant peasant, a lout, the rudest man I've ever met."

But she had already turned against me since her second visit to my consulting-rooms, when she'd asked how much she owed me. At that time I think my fee for a consultation, treatment included, was five thousand francs, which was what I told her.

"Maurice will do you a drawing."

I fetched my son's colored pencils and some paper, and Utrillo did me a typical *"Moulin de la Galette."*

"There," said Lucie, "that's worth much more, but you can keep the change."

But for all that, Lucie can't have held such a bad memory of the "rude peasant." We were no longer in close touch, but in 1955 she sent me a very nice note to tell me of Maurice's death. Her writing paper was engraved with an imperial crown, as were all her effects, ever since a few painters had one evening baptized her "Empress of Montmartre."

I saw her once with Maître Floriot, whom she had been wanting to meet. He invited us to dinner at Fouquet's, and halfway through the meal she cast an "imperial" eye over the assembly and, turning to my friend, the famous lawyer, said: "Now you've been seen with me, the whole of society will hear about you."

I have never forgotten Maurice Utrillo, and often I think of him in his chapel, arms folded, kneeling in prayer. Poor, pitiful emaciated Christ, expressing all the anguish of his life. ". . . Mother, why has thou forsaken me?"

The year was 1950. Police all over the country were looking for Pierre Loutrel, better known as "Pierrot le Fou," the dangerous gangster generally considered Public Enemy Number One. Had they but known it, their quarry was sitting waiting to be shown into my consulting-room, for he was suffering from that occupational complaint of presidents and managing directors, the duodenal ulcer.

He was a small man, with very black eyes and hair neatly parted in the middle, wearing a dark suit of good quality, although his tie was in doubtful taste. I had no idea of his profession, and took him for a successful car salesman. I looked at the telltale lines on his face and his gaunt hollow cheeks, and diagnosed his trouble at once.

"I've tried everything, Doctor"—for so he thought of me—"at least I've tried everything you can get at the chemist's, but I can't stop the pain. It's worst at night, it gets me right here," indicating his stomach. "It's driving me crazy. Do you think you can do something for me?"

I could confidently tell him I could, since I was able to cure 80 percent of such cases. He listened attentively while I told him how he should apply his poultice, his black eyes fixed on mine, asking me to repeat each instruction.

"Can you go on a diet?"

"Not very easily."

"What kind of life do you lead?"

"I travel a lot."

"Do you drive?"

"Sometimes."

"Do you live an active life?"

"Pretty active."

"And do you often get edgy and nervous?"

"It'd be hard not to . . ." He gestured vaguely. "In business, you know how it is."

"While you're following this treatment, try to avoid anything that might tax your nervous system. Nerves count for a great deal in this type of illness."

He gave a slight smile.

"You know, I'd be only too pleased if they'd leave me in peace, but they're always after me for something."

That night my telephone rang.

"It's me."

"Who?"

"The man with the ulcer. I'm having one of my attacks and I've got my poultice ready, only I wanted to be sure I'd got the drops right. You did say eighty? What happens if I add one too many?"

"It wouldn't poison you. Good night."

I never had a patient follow my prescription more respectfully or with more scrupulous care. A fortnight later he came to see me again. He hadn't made an appointment (I realized later it wouldn't have been safe for him to give any advance indication of his movements), and so I had to keep him waiting for quite a time. Nevertheless, as I told him, he seemed very calm and patient for a highly strung person.

"Well, in my job you have to know how to wait. I don't show it, but it eats me up inside." He rubbed his stomach. "I've come to tell you that your herbs really are relieving the pain, so I'd like another bottle. I've got a sister who's taking care of the diet."

He was less careful in his speech this time, and on the way out he gave my secretary five thousand francs, saying: "Buy yourself some little knick-knack with this."

He was back again a week later.

"I've had a bad knock this week; it brought on a real bad attack. Pity, I hadn't had any pain at all until this happened. If I hadn't been feeling so rotten I'd have skipped."

"I don't know what your job is, but it's going to be diffi-cult to make you better if you don't do your share, even if I step up the dosage."

"It's not possible you haven't recognized me. Some guys I can trust tell me it's OK to spill it to you, so I will: I'm Loutrel, Pierrot le Fou. Does that mean anything to you?"

I could hardly have been unaware of his exploits and those of his gang. He was no softie, this client of mine, and his record to date was pretty impressive.

"You see, when you tell me to change my job, to stop liv-ing on my nerves, I'd be glad to, but it isn't easy to lead a quiet life when you're dodging a death sentence and all the cops are after you. You can help me. The guys who sent me told me you do miracles, so do one for me. As soon as I'm better, I'll go straight."

My secretaries thought he was perfect: they found him polite and very agreeable. He came in a different car each time, always a beautiful American model, and they fig-ured he must be very wealthy. They weren't mistaken, for he really was the Al Capone of France. That evening he peeled a ten-thousand-franc note off the bundle in his pocket and left it for them.

It didn't trouble my conscience that I was seeing Loutrel. I wasn't a police informer, and you don't turn in a man who has come to you for treatment. I knew quite well what my father would have done in such a case, and I could not do otherwise. I've never needed to take any oath or make any promises. Of my own accord, I respect the rules of professional secrecy.

All the same, I had a real fright one day when I found Loutrel and one of the top men in the Sûreté Nationale[1] sitting next to each other in my waiting-room. The Sûreté man had not recognized this fellow, quietly reading his newspaper, as the very man whose photograph was posted in every police station throughout France, doubtless be-

[1] CID.

cause it was the last place he'd ever have expected to find him.

I had practically cured Loutrel's ulcer and he'd had no further attacks when he died, accidentally shooting himself in the stomach when he was tucking his pistol into his belt, just after robbing a jeweller's in the Rue Boissière.

The most dazzling man I ever met, and the one I have perhaps most loved and admired, was Jean Cocteau. What I came to treat him for, and cured, was a heart condition— an infarct. But there was something uncanny about the way we met the first time.

There are things that happen to us as if they were meant to happen. For instance, the meeting of two people, both of whom feel that chance had nothing to do with it; that, indeed, it was the work of unknown forces. I believe in predestination, mad as this may seem to some people. What we cannot explain disturbs us, and so we prefer to deny its existence, but that doesn't mean that it does not exist and does not influence our lives.

Mr. Pasquini had told Cocteau about me, and he had made an appointment to see me in a week's time. What happened next was completely unforeseen.

I no longer remember what prompted me to go to the forest of Fontainebleau. Fatigue? Nervous exhaustion? The need to get close to nature? Perhaps a little of all these things, but at all events I had been walking for a long time when I reached the outskirts of Milly-La-Forêt. Entering the village I stopped to look at the château and the floating strands of long weeds in the black waters of its ditches. I had no idea that this was the home of Jean Cocteau.

Everything seemed special to me that day, perhaps because I was drawing near to an enchanter. My meanderings led me to a little chapel surrounded by an herb garden. It was a beautiful day, and here were all my familiar, beloved plants, growing happy and free, breathing the gentle air, the dust of their pollen dancing in the sunshine. I decided to enter the chapel. The God it sheltered was my own.

And that was when I saw Jean Cocteau. He was wearing a rust-colored suède jacket, and his fluffy white hair in the sunlight looked like a halo around his head. He was up on a scaffolding, decorating the walls of the little chapel, and he had his back to me. With every brush-stroke I watched a buttercup unfolding—the very flower I had chosen for his treatment—miraculously coming to life at the very moment I appeared. How can one help believing in hidden forces when the fates send us such clear signs!

With Cocteau, things always became quite simple. He turned round and I said: "I'm Maurice Mességué."

"I was expecting you."

"But I didn't know I was coming."

He smiled. "Nor did I."

"You're painting the flower I'm going to use to make you better."

"How do you know?"

"I use it a lot, and I had a feeling it would be right for you."

I couldn't have talked like this with anyone else, but Cocteau had the power to tune you in to himself. He had climbed down his ladder and was looking at me, and I noticed that beneath his jacket he was wearing a buttercup-yellow pullover.

"I'm glad we speak the same language."

"Oh, I'm only a peasant."

"You're made of blood and clay. You're a solid man of the earth, like my friend Pablo Picasso."

He stood motionless in the doorway, looking at me. He seemed like a bird that has alighted for a moment on the ground.

"Is it not wonderful, Maurice Mességué, that you should have come here, not knowing you were summoned, and found me painting your good herbs, the very ones you are going to give me. Perhaps the hieroglyphics of your prescription are already inscribed on these walls. Come and point them out to me, tell me their virtues. I don't know anything about them, I only know they give me pleasure and I love them for it. Tell me about them."

So I told him all the names my father called them: traveller's—joy, thorn-apply—and that marvellous litany:

> Woundwort and Feverwort and Live-long
> Heal us
> Thornapple and Catmint
> Preserve us
> Moneywort and Pennyroyal
> Support us
> Angel's eye and Motherwort
> Protect us

"I'd like that poem to be sung here in the chapel on the day I die."

"Write it down."

"No, it's already written on the walls. They will sing it for me and I shall be the only one to hear." For a moment his hands were stilled in mid-flight. "I'm not afraid of dying. What I fear is the moment of passing over, but no doubt I shall have some warning. Death is a friend I've so often staged that I should easily find her again behind the mirror. Come along, we'll go to the house. Did you know I'm exactly the same age as the Eiffel Tower—and just as tough. I've an iron constitution." He broke off and smiled. "Tell me I'm still young. It's true, and I like to hear it. I got the knack of 'youth' fifty years ago—all it takes is to be constantly starting something which is what I've been doing all my life. Did you ever hear what André Maurois said the day I was 'received' into the French Academy? 'If ever the day comes when you start to grow old, Jean Cocteau, you'll be doing us all a favor: you'll be starting a fashion for old age.' But I'd say I can leave it for a while yet, wouldn't you?

"I ran into a bit of trouble over that Académie Française business. Some of my friends didn't at all like my acceptance of membership in it; they came up with some big words to throw at my head: traitor, renegade . . . They just didn't understand. People have always expected the unexpected of me, and it was unexpected of me to enter the Académie, so what are they complaining about? The Académie is my latest scandal! Tell me, how do you like my house?"

"I stopped on my way into the village to look at the weeds in the ditches."

"I love those long green strands streaming in the water like the hair of Ophelia. I won't let anyone pull them up."

Visionary though he was, he did not foresee that a few months later, Xavière, his Persian cat who liked swimming in those ditches, would be trapped by the weeds and be drowned.

Just as I had been uncomfortable in Lucie Valore's garden, so this one delighted me. Flowers grew freely over the statues, and gave the nymphs a festive appearance. This was a place where plants and animals, and perhaps men too, were free to do what they wanted.

We went into the house and I examined him. His body was as lean and smooth as an adolescent's.

"I live like an anchorite," he said, "my body's turning to spirit."

Beside him I felt thick and loutish, especially considering that he was thirty years or more older than I. However, we spoke the same language. I would say, "my good herbs," and he would answer, "your wild herbs." I felt attuned to him, not only as myself but as the son of Camille Mességué. In Cocteau I found again all the purity and nobility of my father, which is one of the reasons I loved him so much.

For years, until his death, I used to go twice a week to see Jean Cocteau juggling with words, either at Milly or at his apartment in the Palais Royal rue de Montpensier. It was presided over by his housekeeper, Mme. Racine—Cocteau delighted in her name. If she didn't like the looks of a visitor she ushered him right back into the elevator that had brought him up, saying with finality: "Mr. Cocteau is sleeping."

Cocteau's neighbor in the Palais Royal was Colette, and one day he took me to visit her. As we crossed the salon, Jean pointed out a collection of glass balls on the mantelpiece: ". . . her magic crystals, she looks into them and sees the world." Colette was confined to bed at that time, her gnarled, twisted hands still trying to write on that lavender-blue notepaper of hers, but when she saw us she pushed her papers away. She still had that famous mop of hair, but it had turned grey now. Her nose and her chin had grown very sharp and pointed, but her eyes were still beautiful, lengthened by a penciled line at the outer corners to accentuate the catlike shape of her face. She looked at me as only she knew how to look at a man, and I remember thinking that it wouldn't be easy to lie to her.

"Welcome. Jean tells me you can tame plants the way I can tame animals." She spoke in a slightly husky voice and her Burgundian accent gave a purring sound to her r's. "Who are you, Mességué?"

"A peasant."

"You say that as proudly as I would. You were right to bring him to see me, Jean."

I would have liked to know her better, to help alleviate her pain, but she died a few months later.

Every one of my meetings with Cocteau, right from the first, had something dreamlike about it. His friendship was extraordinary. He "made friends" as others make love. He never failed to keep in touch, and in every letter he wrote I always found words that gave me pleasure and comfort. Once when I was living through the hell of yet another court hearing, he wrote to me from the Cap d'Antibes:

"My very dear disciple of St. Blaise of the Herbs.

"I visited Soulié[1] before my trip to the Cap. He said with a smile, 'Mességué . . . to deny his powers is to value discretion, above all.' And at the end Cocteau added:

[1] The most eminent French cardiologist of his time.

'You and I have the same problems, I don't want anyone to admire me, only to believe me.' "

My treatment, based on buttercup, had done him a lot of good, as he one day announced: "Thanks to this brilliant mixture, I can clear hurdles that would be too hard for plenty of younger men!"

On another occasion he wrote to me:

"Just a quick note to tell you that if I've managed to survive the exhausting work this film has entailed, it's thanks to your herbal baths and the diet you advised. Affectionately yours . . ."

This mildly eccentric old man had a very exact sense of time and—like myself—he had an almost morbid dread of being late. Whenever we went to the theater together, as we did quite often, we would both arrive at the same time as the usherettes. We have even been known to wait on the pavement for the doors to open. And Jean would say:

"Maurice, I have such an obsession about being late that one day it'll make me lose a few minutes of my life. I'd be capable of arriving early for my last appointment of all."

On October 11, 1963, friendship killed him. The death of Edith Piaf was too grievous a blow for this young-man's old heart to sustain.

Today Jean-the-Poet rests, like a great winged insect, a few yards from the chapel of St. Blaise of the Herbs. His soul has gone to join the stars he used to scatter so liberally over his drawings and in his poems.

21

My Great Success: Cellulitis

MY MOST SIGNAL VICTORY has been against cellulitis. Over the years I have cured 98 percent of the cases I have treated. This disease—for such it is—has become the dread of womankind, for of people affected, 95 percent are women.

I decided to declare war on cellulitis, the number one enemy of women today. I had already helped a great many women to slim, but I hadn't really attacked the root of the problem. My diuretic foot-baths—based on greater celandine, couch-grass, field horsetail, common broom, buttercup, ground-ivy, etc.—had proved very effective, and had encouraged me to think I possessed a reliable remedy for different types of obesity and edema. I would perhaps have remained content to leave it at that, had not a young woman, Paulette L., come to consult me. She was small, fair, pleasingly plump, and her pale, limpid eyes reminded me of Michèle Morgan's.

Her first question was: "Do I need to get undressed?"

"No, Madam, of course not."

"That's just as well, because I don't think I'd have dared to."

I wondered what on earth she could be hiding that was so shameful.

"Sir, I've got to lose some weight. Don't tell me I don't need to, you'd understand if you saw my thighs. They're enormous. It doesn't show much in a dress, but in a swim suit they look grotesque!"

"You don't think you're maybe exaggerating a little."

"No. I've brought you a photograph my husband took this summer, so you can see for yourself."

She was right. This lovely, well-proportioned woman, with a rather small bust and slender legs, had truly obese thighs that spread upwards towards her hips and down to her knees. Luckily for her, those were not the days of the mini-skirt, and I remember thinking how mean and spiteful her husband must be to have photographed her in a swim suit.

"We were on the brink of divorce because of this photo. He took it just to be mean. I was perfectly normal when we got married, five years ago, and we went swimming a lot—he loves swimming—and we always spent our holidays by the sea. Three years ago my husband bought a canoe and we spent our month's summer holiday entirely either on the water or in it. That was when I started to get fat."

"But swimming should be an excellent sport for you."

"That's what I thought. At first when my thighs started getting fat I thought it must be because I was developing the muscles, but then one day I pinched myself and I saw that my skin was all lumpy. It was horrible. I realized I had cellulitis. The next year we went down the gorges by canoe and by then I was quite unsightly. That was when my husband took this horrible photo, just to make me ashamed of myself. Now he takes a woman friend of ours down the Seine and the Marne in his canoe with him. You understand, sir?"

"Yes, perfectly, but what I don't understand is the reason for your cellulitis. Do your kidneys function well?"

"Not bad."

"And your liver."

"I have a little trouble now and then."

"Your bowels?"

"Not very good. You see, the last three years, when we were on the boat, we mostly ate tinned things. The only fresh food we bought was fruit, but we couldn't get it every day. Some of the gorges we came down were out in the wilds, and we'd camp at night in little creeks, miles from any shops. It was marvelous."

"I'm sure, but not for your health. You have poisoned your system. Fluid retention and liver upsets are two conditions that have developed largely due to the modern way of living. These functional disorders of the kidneys and the liver, and therefore of the bowels, are generally the cause of either acute or more especially that chronic alteration of the tissues which we call cellulitis."

"I've taken diuretics, and I did lose weight briefly."

"Undoubtedly. But fighting this illness with diuretics is folly. The day a person takes a diuretic, the effect is remarkable. Some people may lose as much as two to six pounds in a day, but the next day their urine retention has worsened, for the kidneys, tired by the enforced activity, grow lazy again, and the pounds that were so spectacularly lost return just as fast. Nor is the liver spared, since diuretics —often derived from mercury or sulfonamides—frequently set up an acute irritation of the liver. Instead of helping the patient to eliminate the poisons in his system, he is in fact being 'poisoned' a little more."

Nearly all my patients set me a problem of one kind or another. Paulette's problem was neither more interesting nor more touching than many others, and yet I continued to brood over it long after she had left. Carried away by my sympathy for her plight, I had said: "I promise you that your thighs will be pretty again and your husband will have eyes for no one else." Now I had to see to it that I kept my word. I was to see her again in three weeks, and if my foot-baths hadn't caused her to lose sufficient weight, what else should I prescribe? If her elimination was satisfactory, how could I prevent her from gaining weight again? That was what really mattered.

I am no scientist; I'm an empiricist who likes experimenting. My reasoning is simple. Those who do not care for me would say "too simple," which may be so, but at least my reasoning has the merit of being clear and leading me to conclusive experiments. Professor Charcot used to say, "Empiricism is the necessary anteroom to science."

I considered the problem of cellulitis in the following way: As I see it, it is the result of chronic poisoning, the effect of a functional deficiency of the kidneys, the liver and the bowels. Therefore, the first thing to do was to get them all working properly, and for this I could rely on my plants, which had already proved their power.

Secondly, it seemed to me that this condition must originate in the type of food consumed. This was what was basically responsible. I would have been breaking no new ground at all had I merely advocated the avoidance of starch, fats and alcohol and put the patient on a strict diet that would make her live on her reserves. This is a depressing regimen for someone who is a hearty eater, although it gets results in many cases of obesity. But for cellulitis I consider it only a makeshift solution at best, because this kind of restrictive diet is treating only the effects and not the cause.

I had three weeks to study the question. As always, when one is tackling a problem, one starts by learning what one doesn't know in order to be able to reject it later. Two discoveries held my attention: calories and vitamins.

It was in 1899 that Marcelin Berthelot discovered that the energy released in our bodies by food consumed is equal to the amount of heat generated when the same food is burned in the open air. This led him to his conclusion that the human being should regulate his daily calorie intake in proportion to the effort he expends.

To put this as simply as possible, calories can be thought of as the coal one shovels into the boiler in order to produce energy. This seemed logical enough, except that coals do not all burn in the same way. There are those that burn up quickly and leave no waste, but that means filling up the furnace more often. Those that are oily burn more slowly and clog the machine. Then there are those which produce great heat and burn quite slowly but leave a lot of clinker and cinders. Not only the type but also the quality of the coal is of prime importance. How about those patent fuels and synthetic coals?

I couldn't get away from this idea of quantity and quality, although, of course, I had become more knowledgeable about various things: for example, that to avoid deficiency diseases a person must consume a certain amount of "energy" foods which burn in the body on contact with the oxygen absorbed by the lungs and are thus a source of energy. These are:

Proteins:	eggs, cheese, leguminous vegetables, fish, meat.
Carbohydrates:	sugar, cereals, fruit.
Fats:	oils, oleaginous fruits, meat, milk and milk products.

It is also necessary to take in "non-energy" foods which contain substances essential to life, particularly mineral salts:

Calcium:	milk, cheese and fresh green vegetables.
Phosphorous:	meat, fish, eggs.
Iron:	meat, vegetables, oysters, egg yolks, fish.

I still had to study the question of vitamins. We know that vitamins are essential to life, and that they are found in every living structure. Chemical research has shown them to be present in raw foodstuffs, and they have been labelled with the letters of the alphabet: A, B, C, D, E, etc. I believe that we shall discover many more.

Vitamin A This is the vitamin essential to growth. It is found particularly in spinach, root vegetables, lemons, oranges, bananas, nuts, almonds, cabbage, mushrooms, lettuce, artichokes, kidney-beans, pumpkin, tomatoes, liver, brains, heart, powdered milk, butter, cod-liver oil, cream, fat cheeses, egg yolk, wholemeal bread, wheat-bran . . .

Vitamin B This vitamin maintains the balance of the

nervous system. It is found in barm, wheatgerm, lentils, cabbage, carrots, spinach, apples, kidney-beans, tomatoes, mushrooms, chestnuts, lemons, oranges, nuts, egg yolks, brains, liver, powdered milk, malt extract.

Vitamin C This is the anti-scorbutic vitamin, and controls the condition of the blood. It is found in fresh milk, whey, meat juices, oysters, oranges, lemons, bananas, grapes, apples, cabbage, cauliflower, tomatoes, onions, lettuce, dandelions, peas, spinach, beetroot, carrots, green beans, potatoes, turnips.

Vitamin D is essential for the healthy development of teeth and bones, and prevents rickets. It is present in cod-liver oil and other fish oils, fish, mushrooms, green vegetables, milk, yeast.

Vitamin E is the fertility vitamin. Its principal sources are fats, butter, margarine, lettuce leaves, oats, wheatgerm, soya beans, corn, rice.

Vitamin K is instrumental in the coagulation of the blood. It is found in spinach, soya oil . . .

This was all very interesting, quite splendid in fact, but I didn't feel I could impose on my patients diets founded solely on this knowledge. The more I thought about it, the more I clung to what seemed to me the elementary notion that in order to remain in good health a person should eat some of every type of food, should have a balanced diet. Above all I was certain that slimming should not entail the risk of any deficiency of energy and non-energy substances, or any serious vitamin deficiency. My studies, combined with my experiments, confirmed me in the belief that while one could attack cellulitis by emergency dieting, to obtain a rapid loss of weight and inches, the root of the trouble still remained. I kept coming back to my analogy of coal: the actual quality of the foodstuffs must be significant, but in what way? And how is it revealed?

I was struck by two facts, apparently unrelated to the problem.

One day my gamekeeper at Marckolsheim telephoned: "Sir, your pheasants are dying."

"Have they been poisoned?"

"No, but they're eating the Colorado beetles."

"Colorado beetles are lethal to them? Why?"

"No, but the ones they're eating are on potatoes that have been treated with an insecticide based on copper sulphate, and the pheasants that have been pecking at them are dying."

I telephoned the Mayor, who stated positively that while this sulphate was dangerous to birds, it was harmless to human beings.

"There's nothing to worry about, the potatoes aren't affected as they're under the ground."

"Have you thought that the rain washes this sulphate into the soil and your potato plants had been drenched with the stuff, the stalks and the leaves were completely impregnated?"

"Well, you know, potatoes are washed and peeled and cooked."

"But what evidence do you have that your potatoes don't contain sulphate? Are you sure that cooking destroys it?"

To me, one thing was certain: chemically treated potatoes could be dangerous.

Another time I had been treating one of my friends, Chairman of the Committee of the Rhone Valley Nursery Gardeners' Association, for extremely bad eczema. He had contracted eczema from spraying his apple trees against various fungus infections without taking the precaution of wearing gloves.

"What it's done to my hands is nothing," he said, "my piglets died of it."

"How did you happen to spray them with it?"

"I didn't, of course. My wife raises a few pigs, and just before the fruit-picking began the piglets escaped, thirty or thirty-two of them I think it was, and they ate the windfalls. Half an hour later there wasn't one of them left alive."

"How do you explain it?"

"It's simple. The fruit had been sprayed six days before and it hadn't rained since. It's all right if it's washed."

"How often do you spray the trees?"

"Ten or twelve times a year."

This being so, I would say it is vitally important to peel any fruit before eating it, which is a pity, for in certain fruits—particularly the apple—the peel contains vitamins that are not found, or are found only in lesser amounts, in the fruit itself.

The very air we breathe in our cities is polluted. We wash in, swim in, and drink water rendered "drinkable" by the addition of chlorine, disinfectants, and chemical microbicides. What's even more serious is that children and too often even small babies drink it too. Cleaning agents, detergents such as are used for washing dishes, are all by-products of petroleum, and are therefore carcinogenic.

The very vegetables and fruits that should be good for our health are actually liable to endanger it. They grow in soil that has been fertilized with chemical manures and washed with weed-killers that we are warned must be kept out of the reach of children and pets, and we are advised to wash our hands well after use. But nobody worries about the fact that these same killers penetrate the roots and get into the sap and contaminate the growing plants. Vegetables and fruits are protected against parasites by anti-fungus preparations and pesticides that too often contain DDT. For years, scientists assured us that DDT was completely harmless, and it has been sprinkled liberally over growing things and animals and people. Today it is known that the human body only partially eliminates it and that it can therefore accumulate to a dangerous level and later cause serious trouble. It is alarming to consider that the food consumed daily by the average American contains .04 milligrams of DDT. Even our oceans are not spared. In 1964 the Director of Public Health in the United States reported the presence of a high level of this poison in the oils and fats of deep-sea fish.

It is staggering to learn that in France one death in five is due to cancer (from 1937 to 1967, deaths from cancer increased from 43,000 to 72,965 per year), and especially when you know that the yellow color of butter is obtained thanks to P. Dimethylaminoazobenzine and yellow aniline dye (O. Amindazotoluene). These additives are perfectly legal, as are the green coloring matter and eosin currently employed in food and in certain medicines. All these substances are carcinogenic in the smallest amounts.

Animal fodder, both root vegetables such as beets and grass (hay), grow in poisoned soil, and the same is true of fresh pasture, except up in the mountains. Everything is sprinkled and sprayed with chemicals. In winter, cattle are fed on synthetic oil-cake with chemically manufactured vitamins. To accelerate their growth so they will fetch a better price, they are injected with antibiotics, a criminal technique employed both on cattle and poultry.

A few breeders in France tried out the effects of radio-active bodies, introducing them close to the thyroid gland in calves, and obtained apparently magnificent and highly remunerative specimens. In 1965, Mr. Travera, President of the European Association of Agriculture and Biology, made a report at the Association's General Meeting which showed that beef treated in this way had already reached the slaughter-house at La Villette and been put on sale to the public.

Even the depths of the sea are not safe from pollution, and it may become dangerous to eat fish. As for herring, the wood with which they are smoked too often contains carcinogenic wood-tar.

The more I investigated, the greater my alarm. As long ago as 1900, Professor Paul Brouardel, one of the pioneers in public health, wrote: "When a man starts the day with milk conserved with formaldehyde, and for lunch eats a slice of ham conserved with borax, and spinach made greener by copper sulphate, washing it down with wine that has been cleared with gypsum and colored with fuchsine, it's a wonder he has any stomach left."

What would he be saying today? Doubtless the same as Professor W. Heupke of Frankfurt-on-Main, who has drawn up a list of the products used in agriculture and the threat they represent to the human body. Wine from grapes treated with sulphate sprays can cause cirrhosis. Fruit similarly treated causes inflammation of the liver, while fruit that has been treated with sprays derived from lead or mercury also induces, in addition to liver troubles, disorders of the kidneys and the nervous system. Thallium derivatives cause balding, loss of sight, paralysis.

None of us is safe from this gradual and insidious chemical invasion. I know as well as the next person that the human machine is an admirable thing and that our system is so designed that it fights swiftly to repel any foreign invader, and manufactures antibodies for defense and attack.

Nevertheless, the extent to which we are all exposed to being poisoned by our very foods is alarming, and for those whose processes of elimination are hampered in any way, it is sheer disaster. A minor malfunction for them can become the cause of cumulative poisoning, making them the victims, among other things, of cellulitis, which in turn may lead to cancer and myocardial infarction.

How often one hears old people say: "They didn't use all this muck in my time, fruit had a different taste altogether, the bread was much better . . ." They are right, of course, and I decided that I would take as my basic rule of dietetics the banning of all chemically treated food, and urge a return to the most natural food possible.

When Paulette L. came back to see me, she seemed quite satisfied: "Just with your foot-baths, I've lost four kilos, isn't that good?"

"It's only a start, and you will put on weight again very quickly if you don't watch what you eat."

"Are you going to put me on a diet?"

"No. I hate the idea—I'm allergic to the very word. It's so depressing. No, all I'm going to do is suggest a different kind of food."

I briefly outlined the dangerous role of chemicals in our food, and she looked at me in dismay: "Then at that rate there's nothing we can eat."

"Yes, there are lots of things. Now the diet I'm giving you is exclusively for cellulitis. Chemicals are largely responsible for your surplus weight, and they add to the weight problem caused by your five enemies: salt, sugar, bread, fats and alcohol.

"You must give up salt altogether for a few months, and after that use only sea-salt, in moderate amounts.

"Be very careful about sugar. Never take more than two lumps a day, and use only brown cane sugar, never the refined sort. Refined and whitened sugar has lost the elements you need for your health and has usually been treated with chemicals. Substitute for it a small spoonful of mountain honey. Up in the mountains the fields aren't sprayed with chemical fertilizers, the pollen is still pure, and the bees don't carry toxic substances. The enzymes of honey aid the digestion, and its mineral salts and acid endow it with disinfectant properties. If the bees have been fed on sugar or sugar-sweetened substances, the label will be marked 'sugar-fed bees' or 'sugar honey,' and is to be avoided. Balance your sugar intake. On the days you eat honey, omit jams, which should be only home-made jams sweetened with brown sugar.

"You must abolish shop-bought cakes. Eat home-made cake, but only sparingly, just for special celebrations and family parties. This brings us to the whole question of bread and flour, which is your number one enemy.

"The wheat now used in flour-mills has been grown with the help of vast quantities of chemical manure. It is pounded and milled by steel cylinders and then bolted so that it no longer contains any bran, protein granules, gluten or wheat-germ. It is reduced to a kind of starch, very nourishing, but totally without vitamins, oil, phosphorus, iron, magnesium and amino acids.

"Flour is chemically treated with gases derived from chlorine or benzol, to whiten it. Another property of these gases is that they kill the leaven-enzymes, the lack of which in our diet makes us candidates for tuberculosis and cancer. The bread is then further 'enriched' with chemical yeast that contains ammonium persulphate, potassium bromate, magnesium carbonate, gypsum, sodium and calcium sulphates and phosphates. The finishing processes are equally dangerous, and culminate in baking the bread in ovens heated with fuel-oil, a by-product of petroleum.

"Bread like this not only makes you fat, it is actually dangerous, as are biscuits made with the same flour.

"Limit yourself to two or three thin slices of wholemeal bread, preferably rye bread, which is mildly laxative and softens the arteries and activates the circulation. In Russia and Poland, where people eat only rye bread, arteriosclerosis is practically unheard of, as are all other diseases of the blood vessels or thickening of the blood.

"In your case, all cereals and farinaceous foods are not advised.

"You can eat a little farm butter if you're sure where it came from, but you must not use cooked butter. Cooking brings about a chemical change, rendering it dangerous to the liver, the stomach and the intestines. All butter, or very nearly all, is preserved by processes that render it harmful to you. As for margarine, derived from vegetable oils, it is industrially manufactured. Oils, too, are put through the same process. In Provence not so long ago people still scornfully called ground-nut oil 'lamp oil.' Those peasants were right, the best oil is olive oil. Use it sparingly and be sure you get the first pressing, cooled to 0°5 acidity, the only quality that can be well tolerated by the liver and that will therefore not introduce any further poison into your system.

"For you, alcohol is poison. Remember that 'brandy' disguises a mixture of brandy and more than 50 percent industrial alcohol. Wines for so-called everyday use contain ethylene acid, monobromacetic acid and sodium flouride, a coffeespoonful of the latter being a toxic dose. Of course, not all wines and alcohols are adulterated. The important thing is not to drink cheap stuff, but make sure you buy a wine from a guaranteed source. Since in any case you shouldn't drink more than two glasses a day, this shouldn't prove too expensive. As for alcohol and liqueurs, whatever the quality, they are absolutely forbidden.

"These are the five absolute taboos, but you should also be on your guard against all types of pork, especially cold meats made from pork. Not only does pork contain a high proportion of animal fat, but it very often contains chemicals (polyphosphates) that are harmful to your system. Buy only from a pork-butcher who prepares his own meats. Limit yourself to plain ham and a little dry sausage. Do not eat any kind of *pâté*, galantine, potted meat, etc. You must not take cream, drink full-cream milk or eat fat cheeses."

I could see poor Paulette L.'s expression changing as I talked. By now she wasn't smiling at all.

"You haven't said anything about canned foods."

"In your case it's better to leave them alone for a time. In my opinion, canned foods have been the cause of your cellulitis. Yet if you know what to look for on the label, they can be less harmful than other products. The manufacturing process of canned goods is very strictly controlled, and if the label specifies that the contents are free of any chemicals, starch and coloring matter, you needn't worry. Frozen foods are excellent, as freezing preserves all their goodness.

"You are allowed seasonings, in fact, I recommend them all: onion, garlic, shallots, parsley, chervil, rosemary, sage, tarragon, fennel, cumin, pepper, etc., and all the spices too."

"After what you've said, I shan't dare to eat anything at all."

"Why?"

"Well, either I'd be afraid of getting fat or of poisoning myself."

Paulette L. had just taught me a good lesson. Carried away by my subject, I had forgotten all psychology. So I finished as I should have begun:

"You can eat as much grilled red meat as you like. White meat is less nutritious, and I am wary of veal treated with antibiotics. You can also eat 'free-range' chickens, grilled salt-water fish with the exception of mackerel and salmon, and all shellfish. You can drink coffee, tea, fruit juice and vegetable juice. There's quite a lot left to choose from. Let me work out a typical day's menu for you:

Midday – Assorted raw vegetables dressed with a good spoonful of olive oil and lemon juice.
– 1 lamb cutlet seasoned with herbs.
– 1 green vegetable.
– 1 portion of non-fermented cheese.
– Strawberries with yoghurt instead of cream.

Evening – Vegetable soup.
– 1 grilled fish with fennel.
– Salad.
– 1 yoghurt and 1 fruit.
– 1 slice of rye bread with each meal.

Do you think you'll be hungry and depressed?"

"No, certainly I won't."

"Try it then and come and see me again in two weeks."

Two months later Paulette L. was telling me: "I'm still getting thinner, it's marvelous! My husband eats the same as I do, and he no longer gets any of his headaches or feels tired after meals. I didn't mention it to you before, because I really didn't think there was much the matter with him, but I was wrong—it was making him grumpy and irritable. Next Sunday we're both going for a spin on the Marne in the canoe."

Paulette, although she didn't know it, had been a valuable testing ground for me. She came to see me once every two weeks, and I would modify her diet according to her progress. I learned more through her in three months than I could have in years with many other patients.

I went on applying my new theory to all the women who came to consult me about cellulitis, but the results were not always the same. Some women lost weight quite spectacularly, others less, and some hardly at all. When I was deciding on the composition for the baths I prescribed, it was of no avail to take into consideration all those highly important factors in women—nerves, irregular or insufficient menstruation, hormonal disturbances—for which I achieved appreciable success, I was not entirely satisfied. What I needed was to make a proper, controlled test with several women, so I could make careful notes of their reactions, draw weight and measurement graphs, all of which would help me to perfect a treatment for cellulitis. I wanted twelve women who would act as "guinea-pigs," and it was of prime importance that these twelve women should come from different countries, with a different climate and a different staple diet. They should be between thirty, when cellulitis generally becomes apparent, and sixty, when it sets in permanently. I had fixed on eighteen days as the length of the treatment.

I had to wait several years before I was able to carry out this experiment. At last I was able to assemble my twelve "lady guinea-pigs," two of each nationality: German, Spanish, French, Dutch, Italian and Swiss. The morning they were due to arrive I was feeling distinctly nervous, for I knew that I was expected to achieve a resounding success and that if I were only tolerably successful I wouldn't be spared. As usual, I kept telling myself what a fool I'd been. After all, I could have made my tests without letting on to anybody; it served me right for being so full of myself. Nevertheless, I felt tremendously confident of success.

To win the battle, I had weapons I knew to be effective: my diuretic herbs and my planned diet. I also had a secret weapon: my anti-cellulitis cream. This was something I had recently perfected, and I had every right to expect great things of it, since all my previous experiments with it had proved highly satisfactory. This cream has the property of dissolving the cellulitis nodules painlessly, which is important, for if massage of these hardened tissues is to be effective it must be painful, so a lot of women give it up. I have also always been of the opinion that pain is a deterrent to effectiveness, since the muscles contract against pain and thereby impede the relaxation that is indispensable to the treatment. Finally, manual breaking down of these nodules causes unfortunate inflammation that can render the tissues more liable to poisoning. So I had decided to use massage solely as a means of relaxing the nerves and helping the circulation, and at the same time of applying my herbal cream, which would penetrate the skin by osmosis.

The cream obviously does not bring such quick results as the baths, but it has the advantage of attacking the cellulitis locally at the exact spots where it has set in. I had already seen that it restored elasticity and suppleness to the skin and helped legs and tired ankles to become shapely and slender once more.

Since these ladies did not leave my property at Mougins, I was able to keep a constant watch on them and make sure they took the baths at the right time and didn't skip a single one. I could also be sure than no changes were made in their diet, unless I ordered it, and that my cream was applied as it should be. They were all weighed, measured and examined on arrival, under medical supervision, and this was to be repeated after eight days and again at the end of the treatment. I would gladly have aged eighteen days overnight, so impatient was I to know the outcome. Any course of treatment can produce surprises.

The schedule was very precise:

8.00 A.M.	Get up, herbal foot-bath for 8 minutes.
8.30 A.M.	Breakfast: coffee, tea with lemon or special cocoa (fat free), one slice of rye bread. One piece of fruit from my own orchard. Rest. Reading.
10.00 A.M.	Gentle, deep massage with my cream. The qualified masseuse, following my directions, concentrated on hips, thighs and shoulders (where the "bison's hump" develops).
11.00 A.M.	Rest and bath or shower, as preferred.
12.30 P.M.	Lunch, consisting of natural foods. Raw vegetables, seasoned with first-pressing olive oil cooled to 0°5 acidity, and lemon juice. Grilled red meat, ideally 5 1/4 ounces, without salt but seasoned with Provençal herbs. Choice of green vegetable with parsley, chervil, tarragon, garlic, onion and a pat of butter. Non-fermented cheese (1 ounce), 1 slice of rye bread, coffee or tea without sugar.
2.30 P.M.	Rest, reading, conversation, preferably lying down. This position rests the kidneys and is favorable to the action of the diuretic herbs.
4.00 P.M.	Face and body care with a herbal revitalizing cream followed by a herbal beauty mask to prevent the sagging tissues that can result from slimming.
5.00 P.M.	Second medical massage with anti-cellulitis cream.
6.00 P.M.	Walk.
7.30 P.M.	Dinner: vegetable broth, unsalted green vegetables, hard-boiled egg from grain-fed hens, or grilled fish with fennel, or unsalted ham, one yoghurt and one fruit. One slice of rye bread.
10.00 P.M.	Bedtime.

They drank a quart of liquid in the course of each day: mild mineral water, natural fruit juice (not too much, because of its sugar content), unsweetened lemon juice for those whose stomachs could take it. No alcoholic beverages were allowed, of course, nor were pork (except unsalted ham), cakes and sweets.

This shock treatment produced amazing results: By the end of the course my "lady guinea-pigs" had lost 230 pounds (more than a hundred kilos) among them. Their waist measurements had decreased on average by 2 1/2 inches (six centimeters) and bust and hip measurements by 3 1/2 —4 1/2 inches (eight to ten centimeters).

"*Maravilloso!*" said the Spanish ladies.

"*Bellissima!*" enthused the Italians, although they had lost only eleven pounds each.

"*Prima!*" said the Germans, admiring themselves in the mirror, as well they might. Mrs. L. had gone down from 191 pounds to 167.

The most interesting cases were the Frenchwomen.
Madam D. from St.–Claude in the Jura, weighed 158 pounds on arrival. Her height was 5 feet (1m 52), her age 57.

"When I was married, I weighed barely 121 pounds. I was a bit on the plump side, but that was my nature, and my husband liked me that way. He liked my cooking too. We were both very fond of our food, and I could eat what I liked, my weight never varied. I was happy. Then my husband died. I was so wretched I lost nearly 9 pounds."

Before long, having no other pleasures in her life, she took to eating as others take to drink. Within a few months she had put on 37 pounds, and since then no amount of dieting or pills or long walks had made any lasting difference.

At the end of her eighteen-day course, she weighed 138 pounds (a loss of 20 pounds), her neck measurement had decreased by 5 inches (12 centimeters), hips and bust by 3 inches, thighs by 2 1/5 inches, calf measurement by 1 1/5 inches and ankles by 3/4 inch. She was unrecognizable.

"When I looked in the mirror, I said to myself, that can't be you! And the wonderful thing is that it's been so painless and easy. I was afraid I might end up looking haggard, with a lot of new lines and wrinkles. But not at all. Thanks to your cream and the massage, I even look younger."

The case of a woman from Limoges was more serious. She weighed 176 pounds on arrival, her height was 5 feet 3 inches (1m 62), and she was 61 years old.

"Just imagine, in 1928 I was elected Queen of Paris. I doubled for Mistinguett at the Moulin Rouge. Fully clothed I weighed only 112 pounds—and look at me now.

"Too much worry isn't good for women. I was married in 1934 and divorced in 1947, when I was forty. That's a bad age for a woman. I was too much alone, I was bored, so I began to eat, and to put on weight steadily."

Her waist measured 41 inches (104 centimeters), bust and hips 45 inches (116 centimeters). Her blood pressure was very high and her overworked heart, suffocated by fat, was threatened with infarction. She suffered from insomnia and was in a terrible state of depression.

She was a fat, watery-eyed, wheezing old lady.

At the end of the course her weight was down to 158 pounds: she had lost 18 pounds. Her bust measurement was was 42 in., waist 33 1/2 in., hips 36 1/2 in., and thighs 18 3/4 in. She had even lost 1 in. on her arms. Her blood pressure was down by nearly a quarter of what it had been, and she was sleeping eight hours a night without sleeping pills.

She was overjoyed, and kept saying, "I'm ten years younger, I feel as if I'm walking on air. You've worked a miracle. I'd never have believed it." I heard a year later that she still hadn't put on so much as an ounce.

I learned a great deal from this experiment, not only that my method was a good one, but also the important part played by the mind in slimming treatment. One of my Dutch ladies said to me:

"Your treatment has done wonders. But you wouldn't have got the same results in gloomy, grey, rainy surroundings. It's easier to do without one of life's pleasures when everything else is lovely: flowers, sunshine, gaiety. Boredom makes you fat." The German woman agreed with her: "These eighteen days would have been hell at home, but here it's been heavenly."

Now I was beginning to understand why the two Italian women had lost 50 percent less than the others. This country had nothing to offer them that they didn't have in their own. They had no feeling of being abroad, it was just an extension of Italy. But, that being so, why had the Spanish women lost as much weight as the women from the North and the East? My question was answered when one of them told me:

"Our country is perhaps more beautiful than this, but we don't have the same freedom. Things haven't changed much for most women. We still stay at home a lot, our husbands don't like us to go about having fun by ourselves! But here we can. Staying shut up inside your house and inside yourself makes you fat."

My greatest reward was seeing them all go off, free of so much excess weight, happy women once more.

But while beauty is as necessary to a woman's happiness as rain is to growing things, motherhood is indispensable. I am always deeply moved when a childless woman comes into my consulting-room and begs me to work a miracle for her, followed by that desperate plea: "I'm sterile."

Providing there is nothing organically wrong, I get very good results in cases of sterility. When my treatment had been successful I began to follow it up by applying my ideas about diet to the future mother. They would come to tell me their good news and ask my advice. Obviously they were in the care of their doctor or gynecologist, but what they needed from me was something quite different. They would ask what they should do to ensure that their precious child would be born healthy and strong. They were counting on me to advise them, so I had to give serious thought to the question of the health of women in pregnancy, although, apart from these special cases, pregnant women were seldom among my patients.

A pregnant woman must safeguard the closely linked lives of two people. It is doubly important for her to keep to a natural diet, as she must see to it that through her the baby does not absorb even an infinitesimal quantity of chemicals. We only have to remember the appalling tragedy of the thalidomide babies.

The slaphappy way in which certain chemicals are employed is quite frightening. It was recently observed that the weed-killers known as defoliating sprays can turn a perfectly normal fetus into a monstrosity. Since 1961 the forests and crops in South Vietnam have been sprayed with 50,000 tons of an American chemical, 2-4-5 T, and in the ensuing years it has been observed that many women have given birth to a misshapen fetus, and that the percentage of deformities in new-born babies has shown an abnormal increase.

In the event of their contracting some mild illness—flu, colds, tonsilitis—I warn pregnant women against the unnecessary use of sulfanilamides, penicillin, barbiturates and other sedatives and sleeping pills. A pregnant woman is often subject to considerable discomfort, but she must have courage and be patient. She must take no pills at all, not sleeping pills or happy-pills or pills to "keep her going." I go even much further and seriously advise against the use of cosmetic creams containing chemicals. I advise them to wear waterproof gloves whenever they are using washing powders, household cleaning agents, or poisons. Since my herbs penetrate through osmosis, there's no reason to suppose that these products would not do likewise.

By safeguarding the health of a mother-to-be we are also safeguarding her child. When I consider how unthinkingly we all too often treat a pregnant woman, with no concern for her baby, I tell myself that the Good Lord must surely be working miracles every day. This child, already more or less contaminated while still in his mother's womb, is born into a society that uses, both on him and his immediate surroundings, many products that are prejudicial to his health. A good many cases of infantile eczema and diaper rash are due to the washing powders used to launder the baby's clothes and diapers. Many of the products used daily for the child are derivatives of petroleum or contain carcinogenic tars. From his food and even from his mother's milk, through his skin, his mucous membranes, his mouth and his respiratory tract, the new-born baby absorbs more or less minute doses of chemicals. To protect him against flies his room is sprayed with insecticides and germ-killers that might well be more harmful to him than the flies themselves, since he absorbs the falling spray. These insecticide sprays are so dangerous that users are instructed to make sure there is no fruit or other foodstuffs in the room. And we let a baby breathe them in! To purify the air, boil some eucalyptus leaves with a few drops of menthol, and let the vapor spread through the room. Far from poisoning him, it will be good for his lungs.

The products with which we tend and nourish small babies today, even the very vitamins they are given, are no longer natural products. Babies are born with a liver like an adult's. They get colic, they get acute rheumatoid arthritis, all because their mothers dosed themselves without realizing the possible harm to the baby. Our grandparents had much wiser ways of dealing with minor ailments. There was no penicillin to take for a sore throat. On every bedside table there stood an infusion-pot, gently heating over a night-light, with a glass, some sugar and a bottle of orange-flower water.

In pediatrics especially, we should use plants, for natural medication does not give a "shock" to the system—that well-known medical "shock" that can do more damage than the illness itself. Plants work more effectively on children than on anyone else, and the results they bring about have nothing to do with auto-suggestion. On the contrary, babies cry when you give them foot-baths, children of three or four yell blue murder when you apply a poultice. A pill is much easier to take. By the time children reach the age of ten or twelve and are imbued with the pseudo-scientific prejudices of our time, they are only too likely to consider herbal treatment quite ridiculous—nothing but a lot of old wives' tales that go back to the Dark Ages. You could hardly say they are predisposed to believe in the efficacy of herbs, and yet they are the ones who respond best and quickest to herbal treatment. I have always treated my own sons with plants. Whenever they were constipated, I never gave them a drastic purgative, merely a spoonful of olive oil and a preparation based on round-leaved mallow and bindweed. If they had a touch of biliousness I would apply a poultice in the region of the liver, made with greater celandine, nettle and artichoke leaf. If they seemed overexcited I would treat them with single seed hawthorn, linden blossom and crimson clover; and for sore throats I would give them sweet violet and corn poppy. When they were stung by a wasp or a bee or some other insect, I would rub the sting with broad-leaved plantain leaves.

This did not prevent me from calling the doctor if they were seriously ill or had an infectious illness. It would never have entered my head to treat measles or scarlet fever with my herbs. I always found that orthodox medicine and my own combined excellently, to the advantage of my sons' health. Moreover, as they had not been accustomed to chemical treatments at an early age, they responded to even the slightest dose, and this, I believe, is an interesting and instructive aspect of the whole question. To my mind it shows up the limitations of chemical medicine. Like Aesop's Fables, it illustrates the good side and the bad.

22

How I Won the Tour de France

ONE HEARS A LOT about women's nerves and their delicate psychology, and far less about athletes, who share the same problems. These lonely men, who must constantly venture their reputation or their titles in one evening in a boxing ring, in a few hours on a bicycle, in a few minutes in a stadium, are subject to nerves and acute anxiety to such an extent that their success or failure is summed up by their trainer or manager in the words: "He's in good spirits," or "He wasn't in good spirits."

The consequences of our ill-regulated diet have concerned me not only with regard to women and sick people but also with regard to athletes. They should be nourished as carefully and strictly as thorough-breds, for the smallest vital element lacking in their diet can have tragic consequences for them. On every Tour de France you see men collapsing at the road-side, doubled up with pain, complaining of stomach-ache, as if they had been poisoned.

And indeed they are, though not by some criminal hand slipping actual venom into their food or drink. The victim has merely drunk or swallowed enough of the chemicals in our air, our diet, to add up to a systemic poisoning that finally twists his guts and knocks his legs out from under him.

Sport has always been my passion. Personally I have participated chiefly in team sports, but I can understand very well the needs of a lone athlete, such as a champion cyclist, at the height of a race. I fully realized that what he re-quired was a diet that is nourishing but not heavy, that will tone and build up his muscles, stimulate his heart action without causing palpitations, and have a steadying effect upon his nerves. Further, it should be sufficiently varied not to become boring, and above all it must be highly energizing but low in bulk.

It was an absorbing problem and I set about studying it sheerly for my own enjoyment, for I obviously didn't flatter myself that anyone would be waiting for me to draw up a balanced diet for athletes. Once again I was up against this word diet, which is almost always used to mean a tem-porary and restrictive program. Athletes are "put on a diet" a month before the Olympic Games or long-distance cycle races, and the diet, is more or less the same for the entire team regardless of their different temperaments and par-ticular needs. An athlete enters his intensive training, know-ing that the regimen might not be much to his liking but ready to accept it, as he knows it's for his own good. Once the races are over, for the rest of the year he eats what he likes, which is rarely what is in the best interests of his form.

What I was after was for an athlete to be able to eat both pleasurably and profitably all year round. You can't build up a champion in a couple of weeks; you can dope him, but you can't improve his muscles and his tendons and his nerves. So I began asking around. I asked trainers how they fed their boys, and what their reaction was, and they all told me the same thing: "They're very temperamental. You can get them to see reason when they're actually in training, you can get them to eat more or less what you want, but when they're at home it's a different story! And if it's been quite a time since they last raced or boxed, you nearly al-ways have to make them lose weight. Fat is our great enemy, muscles that turn to fat."

To my mind there wasn't much to be said for this, since it meant that an athlete's whole system was subjected to two successive "shocks": first rapid weight loss, and second intensive muscular training. Sometimes they were even in for a third "shock": doping.

I tackled the problem in my usual empirical fashion: What should be omitted from their diet? I am not calorie-fixated; I don't like those kitchen-scales diets that oblige you to weigh everything you eat, nor do I like calculated diets, so much of this and so much of that, which make no allowance for the individual. But I set great store by certain comparative tables I have drawn up, such as the following one relating to the potato.

One boiled potato represents about 86 calories. That same potato is worth 400 calories when converted into chips, and 544 when converted into crisps. Where have all these extra calories come from? From the boiling fats or oils in which the potato has been cooked, of which it absorbs 8 to 10 percent. The lowly potato, thus transformed, has become noxious, to say the least. Who would ever dream of building muscles with cooking fats? Especially when we know that these fats, already adulterated with chemicals to begin with, undergo further changes at high temperatures and become practically inassimilable acids. Add to this the fact that any cooking fat used repeatedly "goes off" a little more each time it's boiled, and you can't help but realize the dangers of this method of cooking.

By the same token I would rule out all foodstuffs rich in animal and vegetable fats—oils, butter, margarine, groundnut oil—for their acids are injurious to both the liver and stomach. I would also rule out tripe and offal, which too often can be a breeding ground for bacteria and toxins and which provide too few calories to be worth the risk. Per 1/4 pound (100 grams), lamb's kidneys have a calorific value of 87, tripe 94, ox liver 116. Animal fats present a similarly unattractive picture. While their calorific count is high—beef 771, pig fat 670, lard 850—their food value is practically nil, and their chief contribution is manufacturing unwanted fat. Finally, I would cut out all foods that are difficult to digest and overtax the liver, such as potted meats that are rich in pork or goose fat.

To keep physically at the top of his form, an athlete requires a daily intake of: calories, 3000-4000; proteins 100-110; fats 951, glucose 850–1000, calcium 1400–1600, phosphorus 2000–2400, iron 30–45, vitamin C 130–150 (milligrams).

Obviously, you can reach these figures with any kind of food. But everything depends on quality. For instance, with 3 1/2 ounces of rice you're getting 300 calories, but polished rice loses its vitamins and its principal mineral salts. Refined and whitened, it is coated with a mixture of glucose, talc, silicate hydrate and magnesium silicate, which are not only useless but injurious to health. Such calorie counting is therefore quite misleading.

Even more than the rest of us, an athlete should eat natural, wholesome foods. I based my ideal balanced diet on six categories in the following order: cereals, sugar, meat, vegetables, fruit and certain milk products.

Top of the cereals I place wholegrain wheat, and in no circumstances ordinary flour. Wheat is considered by all dieticians as almost the sole source of muscular energy. It is more a food for athletes and heavy laborers than for people in sedentary occupations. It is an excellent fuel, if it is burned up.

My comparative tables illustrate very clearly what I mean. Of course, they apply only to pure foods and not those that have been adulterated with chemicals.

	CALORIES	WATER	PROTEINS	FATS	CARBOHYDRATES
100g Wheat	332	13.5	10.5	1.5	69 + mineral salts
100g Sprouted Wheat + vitamin C					
100g Maize	354	13.5	9.5	4.4	69 + mineral salts
100g Barley	330	13.0	11.0	2.0	67 + mineral salts
100g Rice	350	12.0	8.0	1.1	77 + mineral salts
100g Rye	335	13.0	11.0	1.8	69 + mineral salts

These cereals all have their own special properties. Maize,

or Indian corn, regulates the thyroid gland. Fresh corn-on-the-cob is a complete food, rich in vitamins and easily digested. Oats contain vitamin D, and are also diuretic and mildly laxative. Barley is invaluable to the nerve cells and the calcification of the bones. Buckwheat is rich in vitamin P. and, in addition to its nutritive value, also has a steadying effect on the nerves. Rye is particularly recommended for poor circulation of the blood.

Brown sugar—cane sugar only—is rich in carbohydrates, but I far prefer honey which, like wheat, is one of the best energy-giving foods.

Jams made from pure fruit and unrefined cane sugar are excellent, preferably strawberry, red currant, black currant, raspberry. Never eat jelly that contains chemical setting agents (pectins and salicylic acids), or glucose grape juice that is one-third dextrin.

Meat is not such a "complete" food as wholewheat, but it contains vitally important elements. I prefer beef, for reasons that are made clear by this table:

	CALORIES	WATER	PROTEINS	FATS	CARBOHYDRATES
100g Beef	266	59	17	22	—
100g Lamb or Mutton	225	63	18	18	—
100g Veal	175	69	19	11	—

Not only does beef have more calories, almost as much protein and more fat than an identical amount of lamb or veal, it is more digestible than lamb and less often tampered with than veal.

Vegetables and fruits contain considerable mineral salts and also all the vitamins essential to the support of life. High on the list of vegetables I would place watercress, for its vitamin C, sulphur, iron, copper, manganese and iodine; parsley, not only for its diuretic properties but because it contains more than 10 mg of iron; and carrots, which are rich in vitamins, natural sugar and mineral salts. Among salad stuffs my preference is for the tomato, which contains phosphorus, iron, silicon and vitamins. However, it is not wise to eat too many raw vegetables or make a complete meal of them, for they do not agree with a delicate digestion.

First and foremost of the fruits I choose the lemon, which in addition to vitamin C has considerable mineralizing and catalyzing properties, but it will lose the latter and become acid and de-mineralizing if sugar is added. Next I choose grapes, which are a complete food in themselves: glucids (sugars), pectin, organic acids (about 1.7 grams of nitrates to every 3 1/2 ounces of flesh), mineral salts (iron, manganese, potassium, phosphorus, calcium), vitamins B and C, and—what is very rare—water that has radioactive properties.

Of course, by this I do not mean to exclude any fruit or vegetable but simply to stress those that I consider the most valuable. The daily diet should include lemon, watercress, parsley, carrot or tomato alternately, and grapes, as soon as they are available.

The originality of my treatment lay in the use I planned to make of vegetables and fruits. I had decided to forget the calories, proteins, fats, carbohydrates, mineral salts and vitamins, and employ vegetables and fruits mainly for their therapeutic qualities. I was still cautious about milk products, which are often meddled with to ensure that they will keep, and in any case, many adults find that milk products disagree with them. Sterilized milk is pure, but while sterilization kills microbes, it also destroys all the vitamins. It thus becomes harmless but also nutritionally valueless. Skim milk, without any chemical treatment, is a healthy and easily tolerated food but low in calories.

	CALORIES	WATER	PROTEINS	FATS	CARBOHYDRATES
100g Full cream milk	68	87.5	3.9	4.6	0
100g Skim milk	36	90.0	3.5	0.1	4.6

Milk products, such as junket and cream cheese, are

excellent, providing they are home-made with milk from a known source. This is why I prefer cheeses such as Gruyère and dry goat's milk cheese, which seem to be better balanced.

	CALORIES	WATER	PROTEINS	FATS	CARBOHYDRATES
100g Gruyère	391	34	29	30	1.5
100g Goat's	280/380	40/60	16/33	15/25	15

Added to which are phosphorus and calcium in the proportion of 500/700.

For anyone who has to make a physical effort, nothing is better than a handful of dried fruit and nuts: almonds, walnuts, hazel nuts, raisins, figs, for they are rich in phosphorus and calcium.

An athlete should not drink alcohol, of course, nor beer, which has the reputation of slowing a man down. On the other hand he should drink plenty of fruit and vegetable juices, and also pure water, coffee and tea. Coffee is rightly considered a stimulant, but it should be taken only in small amounts or it will overexcite the nervous system and can even cause a serious toxic condition that strains the heart. I prefer weak tea, for its diuretic qualities help in the elemination of body poisons.

These were to me the basic constituents of the ideal diet for an athlete, supplemented by my foot- and hand-bath treatments that would be both calming and invigorating. I anticipated using—except in any unusual case—a mixture of hawthorn, sage, greater celandine, buttercup, peppermint, lavender, knapweed and gentian, and I also envisaged massages with a revitalizing herbal cream. My keyboard was ready, and I wanted to play upon it. All I needed was to find an athlete on whom to try it out.

I waited confidently for the first subject for experiment; it turned out to be the racing cyclist Raphaël Géminiani. I was at Clermont-Ferand when a friend said: "Are you still as keen on sports?"

"What a question!"

"Do you know Gem?"

"By name."

"You know what they're saying. He's lost his form! You'd better help him get it back."

That afternoon I saw Géminiani, and I asked him: "Do you believe in the power of plants?"

"Certainly, more than I believe in all those drugs they're shoving into me. I'm only twenty-nine, but my legs have gone. Can you give me anything that'll buck me up?"

"I'll tell you in a minute. What do you eat?"

"As a rule, d'you mean, or when I'm racing?"

"Why, is there a difference?"

"Of course there is. When I'm racing I have to be careful what I eat. Otherwise I eat more or less everything: *pâté*, meat, eggs . . ."

"And vegetables and fruit, and salads and raw vegetables, and cereals?"

"If they're put in front of me, but I don't reckon you can build up much muscle with green stuff."

One thing seemed certain: my task wasn't going to be easy. I started by telling him:

"I think you are making a mistake watching your diet for only a few months of the year. Intensive training isn't what puts you at the top of your form. Your form depends on what's on your plate all year round!" And I quoted chip potatoes as an example.

He looked rather disappointed.

"I thought you got quick results just by using your herbs."

"My herbs alone can't do much for you. But I promise that if you stick to the diet I prescribe, next year you'll be up at the front in every race."

It was obvious that he didn't believe me, and I was getting exasperated.

"You might not realize it, but your whole system is poisoned, which is disastrous for a man who lives by his muscles as you do."

"Don't be cross. I promise I'll graze like a cow."

"For goodness sake, don't do that, or you'll swallow more chemical fertilizers than vitamins! And while we're on the subject, do you know how much goodness there is in celery?"

And I told him: "Celery stalks contain potassium, sodium, calcium, phosphorus and iron. Half a cup of cubed celery contains more mineral salts and vitamin C than the same quantity of raw carrot, a vegetable with much to recommend it. Celery is excellent for the nerves, and the leaves contain vitamins A, B, and C, as well as potassium and sodium. Celery juice helps to ward off arthritis, relieves heartburn, and is, moreover, a very good antidote for alcohol. But eat only the green outer stalks."

"What else, apart from celery?"

"Turnips for their vitamins A, B, C. Peppers for vitamin P. Green beans, which are excellent for the kidneys, the heart, and rheumatism. Spinach contains plenty of iron, but don't eat it if your liver is easily upset. Eggplant including seeds and skin, is good for the bowels. Cucumber contains a high percentage of vitamin C and eliminates water from cellular tissues. It is also the plant with the greatest power of dissolving uric acid. Only don't peel it, don't salt it, and drink its juice.

"Have I convinced you?"

It was all very well to tell him this, but I was uneasy. For the first time since I'd been treating people, I had started from theory. Even scientists can be wrong, so what were the chances that I, armed with only my own ideas, and with facts and figures borrowed from the specialists, wouldn't make mistakes? But then, as I explained to Gem what kinds of foods he should eat, the usual miracle happened: everything became very clear, and I knew for a certainty the part each food would play in helping Géminiani get his legs back.

Ten months later, in 1953, once more the great Gem, he was among the leaders in the French championship race. For me this was a significant success. As for Gem, he was so thoroughly converted to my ideas of eating pure, wholesome foods that he subsequently opened a health food store, and sent me several of his co-athletes. I certainly owe him one of the most exciting treatments I have ever undertaken.

I treated several cyclists, with some success. My only failure was with the *campionissimo*, Fausto Coppi, although things had looked promising enough at the start. Like the others, he'd come to me because he wasn't feeling on top of his form and his morale was low, which naturally affected him physically. Within a few minutes I had him laughing heartily at my tales of Cardinal Angelo Giuseppe Roncalli, Papal Nuncio in France, who was later to become Pope John XXIII.

"But how did you meet him?" Coppi asked.

"Oh, when I heard him shouting your name. Georgel, the Elysée coiffeur, had invited me for a weekend's fishing near Rambouillet. President Vincent Auriol was the guest of honor, so nobody was paying much attention to the plump, smiling cardinal with the roguish twinkle in his eye. Attracted by his lovely, deep voice with the soft Italian accent, I looked in his direction and saw a man with the calm and solid appearance of a peasant, which of course is what he was. I took an instant liking to him. I saw him glance at his watch, suddenly leave the group he was chatting with and hurry over to switch on the radio: "I hope you don't mind, it's the Tour de France." He leaned close to the set, listening attentively, and then he suddenly started stamping his foot and chanting: 'Cop-pi! Cop-pi!' You were just winning one stage of the race."

Fausto was delighted. Like many Italians he was devoted to the clergy of Rome.

"Did you talk to him?"

"Yes, I spent the whole day with him. Once you'd gotten to know him, it was impossible to tear yourself away. The first thing I said to him was:

"I have a sin to confess to your Eminence: I practice

healing, which the medical profession considers a sacrilege."

"How wrong they are! Healing is very Catholic. We priests try to be healers too, you know! How can we forget that Our Lord Jesus Christ was the greatest healer of all? And he was crucified . . ."

Coppi was happy. "What was he like?" he wanted to know.

"Extraordinary. He had the wonderful simplicity of all truly great men. I can still see him at dinner, respectfully and lovingly sniffing a Haut-Brion. 'See what a fine thing,' he said, pointing to his glass. 'God put good wine on the earth for us to drink—' then, turning to the lady seated .next to him: '—and pretty women for us to look at.' Ever since then, whenever I drink a good wine or look at a lovely woman, I feel I do so with the papal blessing. He loved good things. He ate with gusto but also with respect.

" 'I see that I surprise you, Mr. Mességué,' he said that evening, setting down his glass. 'But you see I'm making up for when I was little. My brother Angelo and I would share an egg before we went to school each day. He would eat the yolk and I'd eat the white. It's not very satisfying, the white of an egg, and I've eaten like a starving beggar ever since. I have a healthy respect for all the precious, good things of life.' "

Coppi couldn't hear enough of these stories.

"And did you ever meet him again?"

"Yes, I even treated him. When he left us that evening, he said to me: 'Come and see me. I rather think I need your help.' He folded his hands, which were very white—although his fingers with their thick joints were still the fingers of a peasant—and in an undertone shyly confided: '*Sono troppo grosso.*' [1] When I arrived at the nuncio's residence in Avenue de Président Wilson two days later, he greeted me in Latin: '*Ave Mauricius!*' He'd asked me to come very early, at six in the morning, which surprised

[1] "I am too fat."

me. 'How is it that your Eminence is such an early riser?'
I asked him.

" 'I get up at five o'clock every morning, and I never
need an alarm clock. I just ask my guardian angel every
evening to wake me up.'

"I think that what appealed to me most about him was
his love of people and the way he was at ease with all kinds
of people, high and low. So I asked him:

" 'How is it that your Eminence gets on so well with
everybody?'

" 'That's simple. It's because I get on well with myself,
and for that, all you need is a good stomach, a good liver,
and an easy conscience.' "

"But what did you treat him for?"

"You don't imagine I'm going to tell you?

"At that time I had no more idea that he was going
to become Pope than he evidently did himself. One of the
last times I saw him he said:

" 'I shouldn't like to be Pope, Mr. Mességué, because,
you see, I like to eat in company, and Vatican protocol
demands that the Pope sit alone at table, and what's more,
he's watched over by a dignitary standing behind. It would
quite spoil my appetite, in fact I think I'd likely ask the
gardener to share my meal. Imagine the scandal!' And he
laughed heartily, little imagining that nine years later he
was going to become John XXIII."

I remained on the friendliest terms with Fausto Coppi,
but I met with total failure as far as he was concerned. I
don't know whether he actually followed my treatment or
whether he had a resistance to plants, just as some people
do to penicillin or other medicines, but on his subsequent
visits I could perceive no change in his condition. He kept
telling me:

"I assure you I take my foot-baths and conscientiously
soak my hands in your green herb water, but I'm just the
same. I've no interest in anything, I get no pleasure from

whatever I'm doing. I feel as if there's something missing in my life—but what?"

A few months later he'd found what had been missing, and he entered my consulting-room a different man: "It's all right, Mességué, I've found what it was I was missing!"

I doubted that my herbs were the cause of this sudden transformation, and I was right: Fausto Coppi had met his lady love. Once more I was reminded that a person often only needs to be happy in order to regain his health.

23

Cancer

A HEALER'S GOOD NAME is no more secure than the title held by a champion. Where a doctor is concerned, everyone is willing to concede that *errare humanum est,* whereas those who heal without the proper diploma are expected to succeed practically every time, and if you don't keep up your success rate, then suddenly you're no longer the "miracle doctor" but a quack. That I have been saved from making many mistakes is, I believe, due to the simple thinking and honesty I inherited from my father.

In 1957 I was called in to see Sacha Guitry. His name to me stood for an entire epoch, an epoch which, being a humble peasant, I had never known but which sparkled and shimmered like a glass of champagne. I knew his films, I had read *Roman d'un tricheur,* I treasured his witticisms, such as: "If the people who say things about me behind my back only knew what I think of them, they'd have a lot more to say." I wished I'd been the one to say it, because it so exactly expressed what I felt myself, and in fact I've quoted it often enough in my time.

He lived in a house on the corner of Avenue Elysée-Reclus and Avenue Emile-Pouvillon. The small garden was pointed like the prow of a ship, with a bust of his father, Lucion Guitry, for its figurehead.

From the rather chill entrance hall, the pretty wrought

iron scrollwork of the staircase led up to the first floor where the "Master" lived. The walls were covered with fine pictures, but I was able to glance at them only briefly as I passed, for I am not in the habit of keeping a patient waiting. And I was only there, alas, to see a patient, a patient by the name of Sacha Guitry.

I was deeply moved to see this man whom women had so loved, and whom certain men had so hated. His complexion was a pallid grey, his beard, trimmed like Pasteur's, accentuated a style and bearing that belonged to another age. Around his neck was the Oriental rosary of red amber he wore all the time, like a charm. He plucked gently at the beads with those hands he was so proud of but which now had practically no strength left in them. His emaciated body was wrapped in the brilliant folds of a mauve satin dressing-gown.

For the first—and last—time I heard that famous "Aaah" which preceded everything he said.

"Aaah . . . the herb doctor, your plants will have to work wonders to get me out of this one. Did they tell you I like violets, Parma violets?"

Two long, sad lines ran from the famous nose, which had won him the role of Louis XV (Louis *le Bien-Aimé*), down to his mouth. Death had already started to model a noble mask, and his eyes could discern things that the healthy cannot see.

My visit was too short. The patient was tired, and there was nothing I could do. Lana Marconi, his wife, took me into his study, where I looked at his touching collection of well-lived objects: Molière's inkwell, Toulouse Lautrec's tiny walking stick, Joffre's flag from the Battle of the Marne, plaster casts of famous hands: Cocteau's, Colette's, his own.

"Well then, what can you do for him?" his wife asked.

I could only answer: "Nothing, Madam. You told me the Master has cancer, and I do not treat cancer."

My position with regard to this terrible illness has been unvarying. It would be criminal on my part to claim to cure cancer, so I feel particular anguish at the ravages of this scourge of our civilization. It used to be a little-known and almost non-existent disease, but with the industrial development of our cities, the chemical additives to our foods, the excessive use of tobacco, with air pollution and the steady shrinkage of forests and open spaces, we have seen cancer come dramatically to the fore.

In the course of a single day's consultations, I see from one to five people who have cancer. It is an ordeal for me every time I have to say, "There's nothing I can do for you." I have received extraordinary offers in my time. In 1965, a wealthy olive grower in western Tunisia went so far as to offer me, through an intermediary, a fee of a million francs if I would agree to treat his wife, who had cancer. The friend, who acted as go-between, was to get $60,000 commission. I might say that, however hard I find it to refuse to treat a sick person, I've never found it at all hard to turn down that kind of proposition. How I wish I knew a "cancer herb," but I know of no such plant. I am sure the day will come when scientists succeed in isolating this virus, but in the meantime we have too few weapons against it, little more than cobalt rays and surgery.

However, although I do not treat the illness, my advice to cancer sufferers is not completely useless. Quite a few people indirectly owe their cure to me, for I do not merely advise surgery but almost inadvertently drive them to it. Too often I represent a last hope to patients who come to me, and when I refuse to treat them they are made aware of the gravity of their condition and realize that only medicine and surgery can save them. Clearly, had they gone to someone who assured them that he could cure them, they wouldn't have been operated on and they'd have lost their one chance of being saved. One cannot repeat too often that cancer is curable providing it is caught in time. That I am at least able to help patients to this extent is very important to me.

Recently a young television actress from Berlin came to

me. She was radiantly beautiful, in the way one associates with German girls. With her blonde hair and bright blue eyes and smooth, firm skin, she was a perfect picture of youth and health. But her outward appearance belied the painful truth: "I have cancer of the breast," she told me.

I at once advised her to have an operation. Her blue eyes darkened like a stormy sea, her pretty lips tightened and she cried out harshly: "I'd sooner kill myself!"

For over an hour I argued with her.

"Sir, I have a good figure?" That much was obvious. "I couldn't stand the idea of being mutilated."

In vain I tried to convince her that she would eventually have to be operated on, perhaps too late, and that the removal of her breast would then be inevitable. There was no reasoning with her, and as she left she said: "Sir, I'd rather you had been dishonest, because I'd have gone away happy."

"But not for long."

Sadly she replied: "Happiness never lasts long. But I thank you anyway. The only thing I ask you is not to tell my parents. My mother wouldn't be able to bear it. Promise you'll forget I ever came to see you."

I promised, but that evening I was haunted by the vision of this beautiful girl. I had to do something; there was every chance she could be saved. When cancer is caught in time, the statistics are very reassuring: for a breast tumor half an inch in diameter, the mortality rate is 10 percent. But if you leave it until the tumor measures two inches, the mortality rate goes up to 90 percent. This young woman still had a chance of living for many years. My promise to say nothing to her parents could not be allowed to outweigh this consideration. I wrote to them at once.

I received two letters in reply: an angry one from their daughter, and a grateful one from them. All this happened a few years ago, and I happen to know—for we long ago made our peace—that she is now perfectly well.

At present 2 1/2 million people in the world die of cancer

every year. On average it is reckoned that for every 100,000 inhabitants, 300 new cases are treated each year. Cancer is killing one person in five.

The same statistics show that 49 to 50 percent of these cases are cured, but this is a misleading figure. The rate of cure, as we have seen, depends on the type of cancer: skin cancer cures are as high as 95 percent, but victories over leukemia are rare.

With my Gascon imagination, I see this disease as some evil insect crawling with legs and mandibles, ravaging flesh and vital organs, lurking in wait like a diabolical, invisible spider, watching for the slightest chance to enter our bodies and destroy us. This isn't such a far-fetched notion as it might appear, for we are continually absorbing cancer, breathing it in, and it lives within us.

There are two principal causes of lung cancer: first, the atmospheric pollution due to incomplete combustions of coal and petroleum products. Professor Léon Binet had long been sounding a warning gong about this: certain urban and industrial areas are veritable hotbeds of cancer. The other cause is tobacco. In France alone in 1967, 3503 smokers died of lung cancer, to which should be added cancers of the larynx, the pharynx and the respiratory tract, which have the same origin. About a third of these deaths are due to smoking.

Recent studies in Canada of over 92,000 adults suggest that a cigarette smoker runs about fourteen times the risk of death from lung cancer as a non-smoker. Cigarettes are by far the most dangerous because, for one thing, as a cigarette paper burns it releases carcinogenic tars, one hazard which is not present in cigar- or pipe-smoking. The presence of carcinogenic bodies in tobacco smoke has been chemically and biologically proved. In effect, only one non-smoker in a hundred is likely to die of lung cancer, while out of a hundred who smoke forty cigarettes a day, ten will die of lung cancer; twenty if they inhale. Forty cigarettes a day raises the possibility to 10 percent, and you double this risk if you inhale. The same proportions are valid for cancer of the larynx and cancer of the bladder, which have the same origins. Cigarette-, cigar- and pipe-smoking have the same effects in cancers of the oral cavity, the pharynx and the esophagus. It has also been observed that cancer from tobacco occurs more frequently among smokers of cigarettes with a high sugar content, like American and English cigarettes. It would seem to be less dangerous to smoke black tobacco.

We will have a more complete picture of the risks we are running today when we realize that the presence of carcinogenic substances has been revealed in tobacco, tar, the yellow coloring of butter, aniline, aniline dyes and benzene hydrocarbons, to which should be added the afla-toxin contained in peanuts that are used in the manufacture of ground-nut oils and are responsible for liver cancers, etc. There are about a hundred substances listed as calculated to induce the development of a cancerous tumor.

One's paralyzing helplessness in the face of advanced cancer is hard to bear, and more than ever does one real-ize the wisdom of the old saying: "An ounce of prevention is worth a pound of cure." It is my belief that a sound diet can be a powerful preventive of the conditions that predispose to cancer. One of my surgeon friends, who has performed many cancer operations in a big hospital on the outskirts of Paris, observed that there was no recurrence of the disease in patients who kept to a strict health diet, whereas there was a recurrence from two to five years after the operation in those who continued to eat indis-criminately. His studies were based on sixteen years' ex-perience.

Others besides myself have noted the effects of diet on cancer. I was giving a lecture on the subject in Dakar when a specialist came up to the platform to give his opinion in public:

"Proportionately as many black Africans working among us and eating as we do die from cancer as do Europeans.

On the other hand, black Africans living in the bush within a radius of thirty-five miles from Dakar suffer from all kinds of diseases but very rarely from cancer. Skin cancer is virtually unknown to them, for their natural pigmentation protects them from the ultraviolet rays that so often give rise to cancer. I cannot sufficiently warn all those girls and boys who sun themselves at such length that, years later, they may have to pay for it dearly."

One of my friends, Dr. Renon, who had been a surgeon in southern Morocco, told me:

"In 40 years' practice I operated almost exclusively on Bedouin; in all that time I came across only two cases of cancer. Then ships started to bring cargoes of European food, and as these foodstuffs became more and more widely adopted, I found myself operating on more and more cancers. I am not drawing any conclusion, simply stating the facts."

Evidence like this has led me to ponder the whole question a great deal. I am quite aware that famous authorities on cancer accord little importance to the role played by diet, but I would still like someone to explain to me why the mortality rate goes up when a country industrializes its food products. I am not saying that this is the sole cause. I am simply worried by the evidence. In countries noted for good food habits, such as Norway, Sweden and the Netherlands, the mortality rate from cancer is very much lower, as it is also in a country like Italy, where the people's diet consists largely of pasta and vegetables.

Your diet should be varied. Be warned against restrictions that might give rise to food deficiencies—particularly protein deficiencies, which are too often the cause of certain cancers. To reduce the risk of cancer, eliminate completely from your diet white bread, white sugar, refined, pasteurized, yellow-color butter, margarine, vegetable oils, vinegar, particularly spirit vinegar. Do not eat refined table salt or pork, or sauces and preserves unless you are sure of their contents. Watch out for the words "coloring matter," "essence," "artificial flavoring," for they conceal your most deadly foes. Cut out sweets, flavored yoghurt, carbonated fruit drinks, etc. Do not eat factory-smoked products. Reject any foodstuffs that contain amylaceous matter: look for these words on the label.

The safest and easiest general rule to observe is to eat what is labeled "natural" and "pure." This is still a very good guarantee, for there are very strict controls against misrepresentation. While the authorities may allow, for purposes of preservation and appearance, chemical additives they somewhat airily deem harmless, they do *not* allow the use of the words "natural" and "pure" on products that have been adulterated in any way.

Do not use *apéritifs,* spirits, white and red wine, although red wine is likely to be less adulterated than white wine. Obviously, if you know exactly what has gone into a bottle of wine or spirits, then you may drink it, but in moderation.

Choose natural dairy butter. However, olive oil is to be preferred.

Substitute lemon juice for vinegar.

Eat plenty of fruit and raw vegetables, washing them first, olive oil, honey, fish, shellfish, wholegrain cereals.

Include moderate quantities of meat, milk, junket, cream cheese, eggs, and chicken only if you know where these foods came from.

Cut down on beer, and drink cider only if you know it is really local cider.

Buy coffee beans rather than ground coffee.

Lastly, eat plenty of garlic, which has many properties: it is a recognized antiseptic, bactericide, expectorant, febrifuge, vermifuge, a remedy for high blood pressure and, used externally on swellings, a good resolvent. Its reputation as a protection against cancer, which is not denied by modern phytotherapy practitioners, probably derives from the fact that, because of its undeniably beneficial effect on the whole system, those who have used it regularly and over a long period have a much higher resistance to illness, particularly illness of bacterial origin. In the past, during outbreaks of plague, doctors would place a pad soaked in a garlic preparation inside their mask when visiting plague victims.

In the Gers, where I come from, people use a lot of garlic, and the peasants will tell you categorically that it protects them from cancer. This hasn't been proved, but statistics do on the whole tend to show that the mortality rate from cancer is much lower in areas where a good deal of garlic is eaten. In Corsica there are villages where cancer is unheard of; these are areas where the people live chiefly on home produce, such as corn, honey and goat's cheese, and where no chemical fertilizers are used.

I cannot go so far as to say that if you stick to a sound diet you will never be a victim of this disease, but I am sure of one thing: you'll be running a ninety times greater risk of cancer if you smoke and if you eat any old thing, any old way.

I have often been criticized for choosing the illnesses I treat with a view to getting favorable statistics. This is untrue. I do not want to give false hopes to patients by hanging on to them when they could be effectively treated and cured by the orthodox medical profession. I know my own limitations and the limitations of my plants. I also refuse to treat leukemia, disseminated sclerosis, tuberculosis, and all illnesses that are the rightful province of surgery or antibiotics. Whenever there exists a sure and effective remedy, medical or surgical, for a disease, it would be criminal vanity on my part to want to take over with my herbs. When a patient can be saved and cured by surgery, it would be madness to tell him: "Your hernia will disappear if you take foot-baths."

Unfortunately there are illnesses that nothing can cure. One day I received a letter from a physician in Paris, saying:

"I am sending you two patients who'll be making the

journey specially just to see you: would you be good enough to let me know your telephone number? I'd also like to ask you if you could possibly come and see me the next time you're in Paris, at your convenience.

"I expect our friends, the D.'s, have told you that I haven't been well for some time. I've had Parkinson's disease for several years, and three years ago I had to give up work. Perhaps there's something you can do for me.

"Telephone me one morning to let me know if you can come and see me—it would be much easier if you could, for it isn't easy for me to get about."

I thanked him for his trust, but I had to tell him:

"Unhappily, I have no treatment that could be of any help. Believe me when I tell you how sincerely sorry I am."

Mr. Remy, Advocate General[1] in Amiens at the time, once testified in court on my behalf, as follows: "I had gone to consult Mr. Mességué to try and delay having an operation my doctor had advised. Not only did he urge me to have the operation immediately, but he sent me to a very great surgeon, and even put his own car and chauffeur at my disposal to take me there. That I was operated on so promptly saved my life. And it was Mességué who convinced me of the necessity for the operation."

---

[1] Deputy Director of Public Prosecutions in a court of appeal.

24

My Battle Against the Charlatans

THAT I NOW CALL MYSELF a phytotherapist rather than a healer is not from snobbery, nor in order to take anyone in, nor to make myself sound knowledgeable to my patients. I gave up using the title of "healer," which I liked so much, so that I would no longer be identified with the charlatans who unrightfully take that ancient, honorable name.

My hardest, fiercest battles and most smarting defeats have not been at the hands of the public or the doctors or even my former old enemy, the Medical Council, but at the hands of the healers, the men I naïvely considered my colleagues.

My friend Dr. Claoué was a generous man, and he and Pasquini and I made a fine utopian trio. One evening when the three of us were together, Claoué said:

"Maurice, would you call yourself a healer?"

"Of course."

He turned to Mr. Pasquini:

"Would you call Maurice an honest man? You needn't tell me, I know your answer. So can you tell me, then, what there is to distinguish him from other healers in a court of law?"

"The fact that he does cure people."

263

"Maurice," Claoué went on, "do you think there are others besides yourself who are genuine healers?"

"Certainly there are."

"But you don't deny that there are also some who are charlatans?"

"Absolutely not."

"Have you any ideas about how to clean up your profession?"

"I publicly denounce the charlatans whenever I have the opportunity."

"By what right? There's no use protesting, you have no right at all. And healers like you, the honest ones, will always be identified with the others."

Mr. Pasquini and I looked at one another. I was not at all sure what he was getting at.

"What we need is official recognition of unorthodox medicine."

Here was an exciting revolutionary idea indeed, and the three of us set about mapping a campaign. Mr. Pasquini, who was then a deputy, would propose a bill, formulated for us by legal experts, in the Chamber of Deputies. To gain the support of public officials and the general public, I was to form a group of unorthodox practitioners who would, as it were, select healers worthy of the name and fight against the charlatans. To broadcast our ideas, Dr. Claoué and I would give a series of lectures defending unorthodox medicine against the fake healers.

We must have gone on talking until the small hours of the morning, and after I left I was so happy, my head was buzzing with so many ideas, that I had to go for a long walk to calm down. I could see myself in the golden age of unorthodox medicine, working hand in hand with the doctors and meeting professionally with my "colleagues," the healers, for a free exchange of knowledge, experience, criticism. It was a splendid vision. The Don Quixote in me swept aside all thought of the prejudiced ignorance of the general public, and of the crooked practitioners who, calling themselves healers, take advantage of this ignorance. Joyfully, I walked on in the early morning, thinking my beautiful thoughts, little dreaming that this was to be my only peaceful time in the course of this battle. I still hadn't learned that when a man is ahead of his time, when he declares that "the earth is round," so to speak, he risks being burned at the stake for witchcraft.

We declared war that very day. The skirmishes that ensued were numerous, but all followed the same pattern: understanding from the public, suspicion from the authorities, and total failure with my dear colleagues, the "healers."

It didn't take long to draw up the six articles of this future professional body, which included:

Article 2. By unorthodox medicine we mean the practice of any activity which has as its aim the curing of illness by means not yet included in the definitions of therapy allowed by recognized orthodox medicine. Unorthodox medicine has the legal right to treat any patient declared incurable or who has been given up by his doctors.

Article 3. Anyone practicing unorthodox medicine may do so only when a patient has failed to respond to the usual recognized treatment, and subject to medical advice and diagnosis. The use of toxic products and open surgery is strictly reserved for qualified medical practitioners only.

Article 4. All patients undergoing unorthodox treatment must, in view of the fact that their illness is often of a chronic nature, be periodically examined by a qualified, recognized doctor. Unorthodox practitioners must make a point of seeing that this is done.

Article 5. Every practitioner is responsible for getting a signed discharge note to regularize his own position with regard to the recognized qualified medical authority.

Article 6. Any infringement of the articles governing the practice of unorthodox medicine can lead to prosecution for the illegal practice of medicine.

Dr. Claoué mobilized his parliamentary friends, Cachat, Galmejane, Drouot-L'Hermine, Lecocq. He even managed to get us on a television program, in the course of which

viewers were asked: "If someone you care about were seriously ill and the official medical profession had declared
itself powerless to cure them, would you send for a healer?"
Within a few hours 1325 viewers had said yes, as against
187 who said no.

Blinded by our own faith, and determined to present an
appreciable number of honest and able healers, I founded
"The National Group of Practitioners of Unorthodox Medicine." With continuing enthusiasm, we drew up the sixteen
articles of membership, the Hippocratic oath of unorthodox
medicine, the healers' charter, which rested primarily on
Primun non nocere (Firstly do no harm). The chief clauses
were:

I shall practice my art, and use my knowledge or my gift with
dignity. I shall not gamble with illness, distress, human suffering.

I shall be incorruptible and fair, disregarding the financial
status, religion, race, sex, or any private knowledge I may have
of any patient.

I shall give my help to the penniless with no other reward
than my own clear conscience.

I shall treat only those patients who are incurable or declared
incurable, those who suffer from chronic disease, those who are
officially given up by the medical profession, following diagnosis
by qualified doctors.

I shall never interrupt any medical treatment or delay any
urgent surgical intervention.

I shall refuse to treat any patient who himself refuses periodi-
cal medical examination while he is undergoing my treatment.

Should I break my oath or a single one of these promises, I
shall cease my professional activities and submit myself to the
judgment of those I have elected for the purpose. All this I
swear freely.

As soon as it was known that we had founded this group,
requests began to pour in, and in all the enthusiasm I was
nominated president. A fine job that turned out to be! I
had no sooner accepted than I realized that my group was
doomed to become chiefly an instrument of war against
the charlatans. Attack was the best means of defense if we

were to clean up a profession that evidently boasted more criminals than honest persons. I began to get astonishing letters from men naïvely revealing their "dreams." One, for example, wrote that he had just come out of prison and his boss wouldn't employ him again, he'd been turned down more or less everywhere, but he'd heard there was money to be made in healing so he'd like to have a go at it. As I had been found guilty, too, he was sure I could help and send him some clients. Another, a journeyman baker, wanted to round off his monthly wages by doing a spot of healing. Letters like these were really quite funny, I suppose, but I couldn't see anything funny about letters that said the writer had read the report of my prosecutions and, noticing that I treat neither cancer nor tuberculosis, thought we might come to an arrangement between us. All I'd have to do was send him the patients I didn't want to treat.

I was also sent prospectuses, such as this one:

MD

Homeopathy — Radiesthesia

Predictions — Silicosis, Leprosy, and all other diseases.

Tuberculosis, Cancer, Poliomyelitis, Syphilis, Rheumatism, Loss of Hair, Exorcism of Burns and Scrofula, Dislocations, etc.

By correspondence and on appointment anywhere in France. Our healing powers boggle the medical profession. Come and be treated by genuine healers. Genuine healers have a supernatural gift, they are never wrong.

It seemed to me that they had a supernatural gift for fraudulence of the very worst kind, medical fraudulence.

There are two newspapers that specialize in the publication of little advertisements, next to the Lonely Hearts column, that I call criminal. The advertisers are ready to resolve all your health problems, and they promise you a speedy cure for all kinds of ailments. I have read, among others: "Increased virility by electronic belt." "Cancer, Leukemia, your last chance, apply for details."

Once after a lecture, the driver of my car, with whom I had fallen into conversation, told me that if I or any of my family had anything wrong, he knew of a woman who had the gift. In fact, it so happened he had her card on him, and he slipped it to me discreetly. The wording was of the simplest: "You are in pain, come to me, my hands will heal you."

The same evening, in the bar at my hotel, a gentleman explained to me how he cured cancer by magnetic passes. Out of sheer curiosity I asked him: "What do you reckon it is, a cancer?"

"It's simple. It's a microbe that develops after you've had a blow. It can happen if you bump into something. So, as you don't treat it anyway, send your patients to me."

I was beginning to realize that before we could ask official recognition, my profession needed a good sweep of the broom. It might seem paradoxical that, a "healer" myself, I should take on the responsibility for wielding the broom. But after all, who could do it better?

I had learned that of 40,000 healers in France, barely 500 were "householders" and tax-payers. For the tax-collector, we are classed with the liberal professions, the same as doctors. We may be illegal as far as the Medical Council is concerned but not when it comes to paying taxes! The State officially takes from us money that, according to them, we are not entitled to earn.

It wasn't long before I came up against criticism and resentment. The lectures we gave all over France, Dr. Claoué and I, were undoubtedly a great success with the general public, but they were far from popular with the healers themselves. Whenever I said I denounced charlatanism, I was loudly applauded, and doctors would come forward to congratulate me publicly, but the "healers," who attended in ever greater numbers, would protest vociferously. One of them, I think it was in Poitiers, came up on to the platform and declared:

"If Mr. Mességué is attacking the true healers, it's because he isn't one himself. He boldly asserts that nobody can cure cancer just because he himself is unable to do so. I say in front of you all, this man is an impostor, he doesn't have the gift!"

This was so outrageous that I didn't even get angry. I answered him:

"It is true, I don't have the gift. And I'm glad of it. It saves me from blindly believing in my own powers, from imagining that I'm able to cure cancer, and especially from telling patients that I can, and taking their money for it."

"You see," shouted this fanatic, "he admits it. He can't work miracles."

"Very true, I don't. However, it is incontestable that I have obtained almost miraculous cures, but, like Ambroise Paré, all I claim is, 'I treated them, but God healed them.' "

Attacks of this kind made me laugh, for I was still convinced that the charter of unorthodox medicine would yet see the light of day, and, together with my group, would save our cause. Even doctors themselves had shown their support. Professor Portmann, Vice-president of the Senate and Dean of the Medical Faculty at Bordeaux, had declared in a broadcast:

My position with regard to the healers was clearly defined when I addressed the Senate: on the one hand there are the genuine healers, and on the other the charlatans, who are a considerable menace to public health.

We know that at present there are at least 1500 charlatans. I personally know a man who was forbidden by one of them to see a surgeon. In my opinion the man responsible is an assassin, and I reported him to the Senate.

These charlatans must be punished, and it is not by dragging them into court for illegal practice that we will achieve the desired effect, for this is exactly what they want. What we should be doing is prosecuting them for manslaughter.

On the other hand, it is certain that there does exist between men, between two minds, some kind of interaction that we cannot yet define. It is in this field that healers may well have some kind of psychological influence over the health of certain patients.

The more I went into it, the more I realized that the number of honest healers was very limited, and I adopted a much stronger line in my lectures. I remember starting one of them with:

"Every year healers are killing thousands of patients. I know a healer near Paris who claims to specialize in cancer cures, but since he is inevitably unable to effect a cure, by the time the patient decides to go to his doctor, it's too late. Let me say it, let me shout it out loud: this man is an assassin; he shouldn't be taken into court for illegal practice, he should be up before the criminal assizes as a murderer."

At the end of the evening a doctor, a Faculty Professor who had come to my lecture with a group of his students, all ready to boo me, came up to me and said:

"Sir, I came here intending to trip you up in public, but I was wrong, you're an honest man, and I am entirely in agreement with you. When all other treatments have failed, a patient has every right to turn to whatever means might help him. But only when we have tried everything. For yours is a dangerous profession.

"One of my patients was a diabetic whose life depended on three shots of insulin every day. One day he went to a healer who was bold enough to say: 'Diabetes? I cure it all the time. There's more insulin in my hands than in all your injections put together. Throw all the stuff away and trust in me. In three weeks you'll be finished with it.'

"He was right. In fifteen days the patient was dead."

In the face of instances such as this, how could I do otherwise than agree with the doctors who fight against empiricists? I grew very wrathful as I read the letter a healer in Nice had written to a cancer patient: ". . . There's no point in coming to see you, it would be quite unnecessary. My treatment consists of a special infusion which will wash your cancer out in your motions." The cost of this treatment was 200,000 francs.

At every lecture I was taken aside by the local healers, who accused me of being a traitor to the cause. This pleased me because in my innocence I thought to myself: Good! That's one more I've unmasked, one black sheep less in the flock! I was convinced that I really was helping to clean up my profession, and I prepared confidently for the meeting of my group. There weren't as yet many members, only about a hundred, but still, I thought, a decent enough number and a representative selection as well. I still can't forget that first meeting: it was almost immediately apparent that I was in a minority of one. The gentlemen paid each other a lot of compliments about their "gifts" and their treatments, they swapped anecdotes about their clients, and one of them even went so far as to suggest compiling a kind of guide-book of healers, with stars, of course, all classified according to their specialty:

"So," said he, "under the letter C you would find Cancer. Now we would have to be fairly strict over this, and the same goes for tuberculosis. To be listed under cancer you would have to prove a number of cures."

So there they were, elaborating their plans right under my nose. It was too much for my patience. I banged hard on the table and, trying not to lose all self-control, shouted: "You are murderers, the lot of you!"

The silence that followed this declaration was so thick you could have cut it with a knife. I took advantage of it to continue:

"You're the worst kind of charlatans, medical quacks. I am completely on the side of the doctors where you are concerned. Your place isn't in the consulting-room but on trial in a court of law."

In the next few seconds I heard more insults than I've heard in my entire life. "Swindler! Doctor's paid stooge!

Traitor, skunk, rotter, dirty dog, profiteer, impostor, Judas . . ."

You'd have thought it was a political meeting at the height of the elections. Most of those present had not yet signed our charters, and I yelled: "You'll pledge your word and keep it, or you'll be excluded." In the face of the almost total majority of "colleagues" hostile to this pledge I resigned. I was beginning to understand just how far we'd been mistaken, Claoué and I. The hard core of genuine healers was getting smaller every day. How could we possibly ask for and procure legislation on behalf of men who were self-evident charlatans? The truth really came home to me when I sent a test letter to 800 "healers":

> DEAR SIR:
> Having heard of the marvelous results you achieve, I am writing to ask for your enlightened help.
> I am suffering from a tumor in the uterus, which a biopsy has shown to be cancer. The doctors advise an operation. What is your opinion? Do you think you could treat me successfully? I am willing to accept whatever expense is incurred.
> Yours, etc.

The results were painful; my disillusionment was mounting. Seven hundred and seventeen advised against the operation, promising an outright cure, the price for which varied from $10.00 to $3,000. Among them I noticed the names of members of my ex-group. Only eleven had the honesty to reply that a surgeon was the only person qualified to deal with this particular case. I felt truly discouraged. So these were my colleagues, the people in my profession!

From every side people were writing or coming in person to tell me of their experiences—too often tragic experiences—with quack doctors. I was sorting the charlatans into several types: those who simply exploit patients for money; semi-fanatics who believe in their own "tricks" and accept money or gifts; fanatics or religious maniacs who are actually sure they can save the patient. These are the ones who'll treat anything, though they prefer incurable disease, since they're miracle mad. They'd gladly chop someone's head off, so sure are they that, thanks to them, it would grow again. They are all equally dangerous.

There are some sickening stories of cases handled by these unscrupulous people whose love of money and whose sheer stupidity have turned them into criminals. During the summer of 1958, a young woman of seventeen, Colette M., started to feel perpetually tired and worn out. At first nobody worried, thinking it was because she was growing or overdoing things, but by November 8 her parents were becoming sufficiently alarmed by her condition to send her to the Hospital for Sick Children in Paris for tests. The diagnosis hit them like a death sentence. It was: Colette has leukemia. She has only a few more months to live. In their summer holiday snapshots, she is laughing, so pretty with her dark eyes and chestnut hair, but these are already only memories, for her shining mop of hair is dulled now and her eyes have lost their brilliance.

Her father, despairing of orthodox medicine, thinks of the miracle-workers, the people whose occult art goes back to the mysterious darkness of the Middle Ages, when all things were possible. He goes to see four healers in succession. The first, for $10.00, gives him poultices of magic clay. He pays the same fee to the next one for some suppositories. The last two specialize in long-distance treatment, using photographs. For this, Mr. M.—who is a humble working man—somehow rakes together $100.00 for each. He would have given more to save his daughter. His little Colette dies on March 25, 1959.

Madam G. wrote to me from Lyon:

Dear Sir:

To help you in your campaign against the fake healers I authorize you to read this letter at your lectures.

My husband, who'd fought in the Algerian war, complained one morning of violent pain in his head. At first he tried several different pain-killers, but none of them did any good, so he went to a doctor who told him that he had a slipped disk and that his pains would go away as soon as it was put back. I couldn't understand why my husband wouldn't believe him. "He's hiding something from me," he said, "a slipped disk can't cause this kind of pain," and he kept saying, "it's enough to drive me mad." So he went to see a local healer. When he came home he didn't say a word, he kissed us all, the children and me, and then he locked himself in the bedroom and shot himself in the head.

I found out later that this criminal told him: "You have a tumor on the brain, but I can work miracles with my remedy, I'll pull you through. In a few days you'll be cured."

The tragedy of it all is that my husband believed in his diagnosis but not in his cure. That charlatan killed him.

But this was nothing compared with the responsibility a certain Naessens took upon himself. I first met him some fifteen years ago, when he came to me and said:

"I've come to you in my capacity as doctor of the faculty of (some Belgian town I don't recall). I specialize in cancer, my researches are already very advanced. Do you treat this disease yourself?"

"No. It would be madness for me to do so."

"Then what do you do with a cancer patient?"

"I refer him to his doctor, or if he doesn't have a doctor, I send him to a surgeon."

"In that case we can work together. You can send your patients to me—we'll split the fee of course—and in return I can send you patients who'd benefit from your treatments."

I took a profound dislike to the man. His handshake was limp and lukewarm. Somehow he put me in mind of a tapeworm; he had a face like a tapeworm. I had the sudden feeling that this man was worse than a charlatan; he was an out-and-out villain—or if he wasn't yet, he soon would be. I felt in my bones that he had no conscience at all, that he wouldn't scruple to gamble with serious illness, where the big money was to be made.

I told Naessens that my ideas concerning cancer were

very conservative and that I relied on surgery and the current orthodox methods of treatment.

He didn't stay even ten minutes, for it was apparent that I was no longer of any interest to him. I would have forgotten all about him had I not read in the newspapers in December 1963 that he had set up practice in Corsica, at Prunete near Bastia, where he was treating cancer, and especially leukemia, with a serum called Anablast, supposedly his own discovery. I saw again the contemptible, slimy expression on his charlatan's face, and I knew for certain that this man was a dangerous criminal.

According to the articles I read, the man wasn't a qualified medical doctor as he'd told me, but self-taught, and, as usual, whenever it was a question of unqualified medical research, they even dragged Pasteur into it! I might have laughed if I hadn't been so aware of the hideous results of this kind of quackery. The fear of cancer and leukemia is so great that even intelligent people lose their heads and are extraordinarily credulous about every new wonder drug. We hope so much that one day we'll have effective weapons against this disease that we are ready to believe anything, and Naessens knew this and turned it to his own gain.

I was so sure that he was nothing but scum that I wanted to denounce him publicly. In January 1965 I went to Corsica to see what was going on and gave a lecture to make my views known. I was appalled at what I found, and deeply angered. Ambulance and cargo planes from all over the world were landing near Bastia, and their cargoes of children with leukemia were taken by cars and ambulances to their "savior." It was a fearful sight, this procession of dying children with huge eyes in their transparent little faces, and parents, some of whom had ruined themselves in the hope that their child might be saved. They came from everywhere, and I remember being particularly touched by two of the fourteen children from England: Edward Burke from Blackpool, who was brought by police helicopter, and

Barney Shenton, who was only seven years old and whose expression I have never been able to forget. A special plane had been chartered to bring fifty young leukemia patients from Argentina. It was madness.

Naessens would unhesitatingly produce for anyone's inspection a young man of sixteen, Bernard Ferran, whom he called his "little miracle cure." If my mind dwells on Bernard it is because at sixteen a boy is well past the age of childish delusions and fully aware of the seriousness of his condition. All that bragging and boasting about him was utterly revolting. In Corsica this scoundrel was regarded as a great man, a true genius, a savior of humanity, and this is understandable, for such a golden age had never been known in and around Prunete. The hotels were full to overflowing, the smallest room brought in money. The leukemia patients were wasting away, but the local inhabitants were prospering.

In Ajaccio I delivered my lecture against charlatanism and strongly voiced my opinion of Naessens. I thought I was going to be lynched. They're a hot-blooded lot in Corsica, and to criticize and attack Naessens was to insult the whole of Corsica. I had to be given police protection when I left, and, followed by the hostile, booing crowd, I caught my plane, unable even to collect my suitcase from the hotel.

I continued to keep a close watch on the situation, however, and friends in Corsica kept me regularly informed of the activities of the fake therapist. A few days after I had left, Professor Denoix was sent to Prunete by the Public Health Office and he had a long talk with Naessens, whose overwhelming conceit could make quite an impression.

Everyone seemed to have forgotten that this charlatan had been convicted in 1956 for illegally practicing medicine. As for his serum, it had been in existence since 1950 and had been made commercially in Switzerland under the name GN 24, but was withdrawn from sale within a very short time.

Professor Denoix decreed that, pending the result of the inquiry, Naessens should accept no new patients but continue only with those already undergoing his treatment. Then things really began to warm up. Those who were arriving didn't want to leave, prices went up and up, and the hapless patients all kept on trying to get treatment regardless of the decree, offering Naessens fortunes he didn't have time to take. Professor Denoix had made out his report to Mr. Marcellin, then the Public Health Officer, and it was final: "Naessens is mistaken, Anablast is valueless."

My friends wrote that there had been demonstrations in Corsica on behalf of Naessens, more than 4000 people raging against the legal authorities in favor of the charlatan. But this didn't prevent Naessens from being found guilty, on February 3, 1964, of the illegal practice of medicine and pharmacy. That was one of the times when I, who have so often been the target of the thunderbolts of justice, was glad to see them striking their target.

One year later there wasn't a single leukemia patient "treated" by Naessens still alive.

In May 1965 Naessens was sentenced to pay the maximum penalty, namely a fine of $3,600. It wasn't much to pay for the death of so many innocents.

25

Dura Lex Sed Lex

Twenty-one times my name has been called in the law courts: ten times in a court of appeal, and eleven times I have stood up before a Court of Summary Jurisdiction. I knew the ritual as well as a priest knows the order of mass, but I could never get used to it. For a week before each hearing I was on edge, pacing back and forth like a caged beast. Indeed, to me, being taken into court was like going into a cage, to be imprisoned by the bars of the law, a law which, however lenient, was unfailingly and relentlessly applied to me.

There was no use telling myself that each case was a victory. This neither soothed nor satisfied me, for it was not the kind of victory I was after. I never went before a court without thinking enviously of my father, whose humble way of life was still to me the unattainable ideal. But while I continued to be agitated by the same feelings each time, all the hearings were different, for there was always a dominating factor that lent each one its special character.

The first time I was taken to court was in 1949, in Nice: The second, in 1950, in Paris; and the third, on March 13, 1951 in Lyon: one each year. The Medical Council must have thought I couldn't hold out for long at that rate, but such persecution only brings out the fighter in me. Assisted by my friend Mr. Pasquini, Mr. Maurice Garçon of the

Académie Française had agreed to conduct my defense,
although it was actually through a misunderstanding that
he had originally accepted. When he was told about me, he
had immediately taken my case because to him being a
healer was synonymous with mysterious powers. He thought
I possessed a gift, whereas all I possessed was my plants;
my treatment was far too straightforward for this lover of
the occult. He himself was the highly esteemed author of
several works on sorcery, and his home in Paris housed a
collection of documents about black magic and white magic
that he had shown me and, thinking me more or less initi-
ated into such arts, had asked:

"To what power do you attribute your gift?"

"To the power the Good Lord put in plants."

I knew he was disappointed, but it didn't keep him from
conducting my defense both ably and intelligently. In Lyon,
the city of black masses, he must have dreamed of some
kind of medieval courthouse scene; instead, his client turned
out to be an ordinary fellow with no mystery about him.
Nevertheless, I remember the case as one of the most astonishing in my career as a man found habitually guilty of
healing. As on previous occasions, nobody denied that I
had actually cured people, but I was charged with having
done so! It must certainly have been one of the rare times
that a public prosecutor came into court to testify on behalf
of the accused rather than plead for the prosecution. Everyone was waiting to hear the testimony of Mr. Alexis Thomas,
the Advocate General[1] of Lyon. A leading figure in the legal
world, he had been charged with the prosecution of Charles
Maurras, and the court fell silent when he entered the witness box:

"You see me here, instead of in my customary place in
a courtroom, because I refuse to plead against Maurice
Mességué, who cured me of a liver disease when I had
been given up by the orthodox medical profession."

A prosecution lawyer defending the accused is not exactly

[1] Deputy Director of Public Prosecution in a court of appeal.

a common occurrence but undeniably a dramatic show of courage. Yet I was found guilty, as was to be expected. However, a leading Paris daily carried the following headline next morning: "THE CONVICTION OF MAURICE MESSEGUE CONSTITUTES A VICTORY FOR THE HEALERS." In his summing-up, the judge stated that the findings of the court were that as I undeniably cured people I could not be prosecuted for charlatanism, and he had expressed his regret that no meeting ground had yet been found between orthodox medicine and the healers.

Everyone around me was delighted, but it gave me only luke-warm satisfaction. This is not the kind of triumph I want.

It was all very well being acclaimed right and left every time I came out of court, but I continued to feel uneasy and at a disadvantage. While the courts did much toward making me so well known, they also stuck me with the label "illegal" and this is something that has always gone against my grain.

My latest hearing to date, in Grasse on May 6, 1968, was certainly the most important, both for me and for unorthodox medicine. Nothing was missing: letters from judges, 220 testimonials from doctors, and about 20,000 moving testimonials from patients, and even a supporting statement from a professor of medicine. For the first time the proceedings went beyond the person of Maurice Mességué and at last touched the fundamental problem.

The proceedings were opened by a seventy-year-old professor of medicine and pharmacy:

"In the house of the accused we seized several large containers that held the preparations he was prescribing for his patients."

He then went on to say that he and his colleagues had tried the contents on dogs. This was too much, and I broke in with: "But I'm not a vet! It was easy for you, Professor, to question me, to ask for my notes, as well as all the notes I have from the two thousand doctors who have sent me patients to date. But why did you not conduct your tests on humans?"

The professor didn't even glance in my direction. His dry hands resting on the bench like the claws of a bird, he gave a slight shrug of his bony shoulders.

President Préau was not convinced.

"Professor," he said, "perhaps there is no scientific proof that Mr. Mességué cures people, but it must be acknowledged that many patients, after following his treatments, consider that they are cured. So, then, to what do you attribute these results?"

"Naturally, patients who follow treatment ordered by their doctor and who also have confidence in Mességué are likely to be cured."

The professor continued:

It's simple, Mr. President. There are three possibilities. One, the patient wasn't really sick, he only thought he was sick; perhaps his doctor also (*errare humanum est*) thought he was sick. Mességué treats him, the imaginary illness disappears. The testimonies of both patient and doctor are valueless, inasmuch as Mr. Mességué has cured a man who was perfectly healthy.

In the second case, the patient is genuinely sick and has been under medical treatment for a long time. He believes the treatments are not working, so he goes to Mr. Mességué, who prescribes foot-baths, which coincide with the precise moment the remedies he'd taken previously began to take effect. Mr. Mességué gets the credit, but the way I see it, he's only cured a patient who was virtually cured already.

In the third case, the patient is a psychopath. This is the kind of patient you treat with placebos—give them a sugar-coated bread-crumb and they'll feel better next day. Foot-baths or hand-baths play the same role. Mr. Mességué is unwittingly practicing psychosomatic medicine: he's cured a man who had virtually nothing wrong with him.

President Préau was not satisfied.

"How is it then, Professor," he continued, "that you didn't think of questioning the patients who claim they were cured? In my opinion you should have examined them yourself."

"There wasn't time, Mr. President, there are too many of them."

"You could have gotten in touch with Mr. Mességué and questioned him."

The professor drew himself up.

"Mr. President, do you believe that in this day and age, when legitimate science has almost mastered the problems of hormones and allergies, when reason and logic have led to the discovery of antibiotics and anesthetics, when we're making enormous headway in transplants—do you think that in the age of the electron microscope there is truly anything to be gained from a study of Mr. Mességué's folklore experiments?"

Nothing and nobody, not even Mr. Pasquini, could have held me back then. I leaped to my feet.

"My folklore, Professor, has been the means of saving patients who, in spite of all your advances in medical knowledge, had reached the point where suicide seemed the only certain way out of their troubles."

The professor made no reply, so we could move on to the witnesses. First to be called were the witnesses for the prosecution, but that didn't take long, as there weren't any! You could hardly count the detective who stated: "Being commissioned to collect evidence I searched the home of the accused and seized several plastic containers 4 3/5 inches high and approximately 5 4/5 inches wide."

They then called the witnesses for the defense. I don't think I have ever been surrounded by more or better witnesses than on that day. Before they were heard, Mr. Pasquini opened the proceedings by reading out some letters, such as the letter from Mrs. Bailly, who superintended one of the biggest pharmacies in Paris, the only one with a complete herbalists' department:

"After trying innumerable ineffectual medical remedies, for the last three and a half years, I have been treated by

Mr. Mességué. I suffered from chronic bronchitis and was further troubled by a slipped disk as a result of having lost a great deal of weight. At times the pain was unbearable, the more so as I also had terrible cellulitis in both my legs. I began to feel a distinct improvement almost at once, and today I am once more able to lead a normal life and cope with the strains of my job.

"I shall be eternally grateful to Mr. Mességué. His plants have made a new person of me and enabled me to enjoy life once again."

This was followed by several moving testimonies from doctors.

But the letter that caused the greatest sensation was from President Antoine Pinay:

"Maurice Mességué, who was introduced and recommended to me by a high-ranking official in the *départmente* of the Seine, brought about a great improvement in the health of one of my relatives. She had suffered for years from extremely painful arthritis, and none of the doctors she consulted had been able to relieve the pain or hold out any hope of improvement."

This was the testimony of a man of integrity, a man who didn't stop to consider whether such a gesture might be in keeping with his position, might lay him open to criticism. He made it because he thought it was his duty to do so. The dictates of his own conscience mattered more to him than any motives of self-interest or self-advancement.

Three doctors, two men and a woman who were clients of mine, followed in succession. The woman doctor, in particular, was most outspoken! "Science is a very fine thing, but it has its limits. For all my diplomas, it wasn't I who was able to cure my daughter of her eczema, it was Mr. Mességué."

As the doctors gave their testimonies, I felt that the professor was steadily losing his advantage. Obviously, I have always followed my hearings with the closest attention, but this time I was more profoundly affected than ever before, sensing that this was to prove such an important case for me. The last doctor to be heard was the surgeon Kreps, professor at Basel University:

"As a representative of classical medicine, I testify without shame, although not, I admit, without envy, that Maurice Mésségué's treatments are successful in fields where our present knowledge does not lead to any appreciable success on our part.

"In the name of the legislation of your country, doctors see it as their duty to take proceedings against Mr. Mésségué. It might be their duty, but justice cannot be one-sided, and it is my duty to tell you that this man"—pointing to me—"this man cured my own wife, who had always suffered from chronic asthma, against which we were powerless."

"Your testimony, Professor Kreps, does you credit," said President Préau.

When Lafargue, the public prosecutor, rose to his feet, he delivered his indictment with neither eloquence nor conviction: ". . . It is certainly possible that Mésségué has helped, even cured, many patients. Nevertheless, by his own admission, he has administered medical treatment without holding a doctor's diploma. However, as there are no grounds for believing that his actions have been harmful, I ask merely that the law be applied with leniency."

When the President called upon the defense to speak, Mr. Pasquini rose to his feet. Without oratory, without any purple passages, his face still registering his emotion at the previous testimony, he gave the proceedings their true significance: "You will say, Mr. President, that it is not your job to create laws but to apply them. My reply to this, Your Honor, is that in the course of history the courts —much to their credit—have sometimes stimulated the reform of an outdated law. It may be that you hold in your hands, by the sentence you pronounce, the future of free medicine, indeed of all medicine."

Court was adjourned, according to custom, for President

Préau to consider his verdict. I knew and felt in my bones that this case was the grand finale of my legal fireworks. I suppose I should have been happy, but I wasn't. At a moment when other men might have been swigging champagne, I was filled with a feeling of great weariness. The night was fragrant with the scent of herbs, filled with the sound of cicadas, and I tramped about dejectedly for hours.

Yet that day I even made my peace with the Medical Council. They were no longer against me. The doctors I had worshipped as a child in Gavarret were holding out the hand of friendship to me. People believed in me, that much was certain. But the road would always be blocked by the barrage of legality, that wall before which I would always be helpless.

Such were my thoughts that night, but the next morning the newspapers were shouting "Victory!" and the headlines ran: THE GRASSE CASE: THE STARTING POINT FOR A LIBERATED MEDICINE and SINCE THE HEALER HEALS, ACQUIT HIM!

The court didn't go as far as to do that, but their sentence, returned on May 6, carried the following qualifying remarks: "A sentence does not take into account the scientific value of a medical treatment. Nevertheless, we recognize that on many occasions Mességué has achieved truly surprising cures." And I was fined only 1,000 (current) francs, less than half of the 2,400 francs minimum stipulated by the law (the maximum being 12,000 francs). All the same, I was found guilty, as I still am and always will be.

It's always risky to predict the future, but even so I think that the hearing in Grasse may well prove to have been my last. The regularity with which I have appeared in court as the accused has surely earned me a break. I think that the judges, many of whom have become my friends, are weary of prosecuting me, of always finding a healer guilty because he heals.

Things have changed since then, and the Medical Council and I are now on very good terms. They dragged me through the mire for twenty years, but now their own lawyer, Mr. Mouquin, appears with me in television discussion programs. In April 1969, the Council for International Cultural Relations organized a debate in which I was opposing the motion proposed by Mr. Mouquin. For me this was a confrontation of great importance, the first ever if its kind. At last I was able to put my point to a representative of the Medical Council other than in a law court, and that day it wasn't I who attacked the Council but one of its own members, Dr. Cherchève:

"As soon as a man departs from the beaten track he is called a healer, he's illegal, he suspect. Remember that Laënnec himself was struck off the register, that Claude Bernard was never admitted to the Academy of Medicine, that Pasteur had endless trouble. As for Freud, were he to come back, to earth today, he'd be considered a healer of the worst kind, nothing more than a "charlatan."

Then Dr. Cherchève quoted this statement by the academician Louis Armand: "Today, whether a man be an engineer, an architect or a doctor, techniques are changing so fast that by the time he's finished his studies he knows absolutely nothing. He's the same as an apprentice plumber starting to learn his trade armed only with a monkey wrench and a hammer. This is particularly true of medicine," he concluded. "To start with, all we have is what is in us. There will be great doctors, just as there will be great healers, according to each man's own personality. Mr. Mességué has said: 'Medicine is not a science but an art,' and I agree with him entirely.

"We reproach healers for their empirical methods, as if medicine itself were not founded on empiricism! The first time digitalis was administered to a man, nobody knew for certain whether it would kill him or improve his heart. The first time a patient was vaccinated, it was the same . . ."

I may not be legally safe from prosecution, but morally I believe I am. I can hardly see the lawyer of the

Medical Council, who has publicly acknowledged my integrity, publicly setting himself against me. Besides, my whole life has been a paradox. While the Medical Council was taking legal action against me, its members were sending me patients and begging me to treat them. To me the Council has never really represented the doctors. With the Council my relations were always accuser versus accused, but with the doctors themselves it was quite different: there has always been a human bond between us. We are all equally members of that breed of men and women who are dedicated to the curing of disease, and for whom care of the sick takes precedence over everything else. Even at the times when I was most persecuted I have always had the constant support of doctors who continued to believe in me and send me patients. They also do so because they know I am a cautious man: I say, "I'll try to make you better" and never "I will cure you." But it is incontestable that I have brought about cures.

Obviously I could not have succeeded every time; I have had my failures. But I have not been responsible for anyone's death, and I also have the satisfaction of being able to say that I have never worsened anyone's condition. Some may say, as I hear they do, "That Mésségué is a shrewd character, he never takes on anything serious. It depends on what is considered serious. Disorders of the circulation or the digestion, rheumatism, neuritis, eczema, asthma and obesity might not necessarily endanger a man's life, but they can be a lifelong handicap, and serious enough for the patient. Surely what I do every day to lessen pains that may not be mortal, but are galling enough to make the patient sometimes wish they were, has its usefulness?

Every day doctors are devoting themselves to saving life, and very often they succeed. It is perhaps because they are ruled by these responsibilities and weighty considerations that they have less time to give to the "little things."

Does this mean that it is not useful for me to make my daily contributions?

I prefer by far to be the healer of these "unimportant diseases" than a charlatan of serious illnesses.

Epilogue

I LOVE TRAVELING, but I love my little corner of the Gers far more. To walk through the woods and the countryside is as good as a blood transfusion to me. When my lungs breathe in the oxygen of that pure country air, then a richer, fuller blood flows through my arteries, and I thank the Good Lord for giving me this love of my corner of the earth. It has saved me from many errors. Success is a frightening thing. Obviously I am no saint, and I have often been understandably filled with foolish pride, but the fact that I am wholly at ease only in my own country has curbed my ambition. I often think back over my life and try to fathom how I came to travel the road from my village to celebrity. I believe the reasons are very simple: luck, intuition, and the fact that I've always kept my feet on the ground.

Intuition has often told me which path to follow, and the firm grip of my feet have kept on the ground has prevented me from straying. When I reach a crossroads and one way seems easier and shorter than the other, I always choose the harder but surer way.

I have never believed that success comes easily, and I have always had the greatest admiration for successful people who lived in fine houses, for I would say to myself, rather naïvely: He must have worked hard to have such success. I have always been fascinated by men who work their way up in life—men like "my President" or Monsignor Roncalli, the little Italian peasant who became Pope. The kind of success that falls to the sons of the rich has never interested me, for there was nothing I could learn from it, no example to follow, no lessons to remember.

In making my way, I have had the usual kind of hardships, for as my father used to say. "It's easier to learn to walk on a carpet than it is on beaten earth. You're less likely to fall, and when you do, it doesn't hurt so much." Whenever I started dreaming ("When I grow up I'll be a famous doctor and I'll be invited to the château"), he would warn me: "Little one, it's easier to sit at a rich man's table than to sit at the Good Lord's. But when you sit at the poor man's table, then you're getting close to Him." No doubt these words account for the fact that the door of my consulting-room has always been wide open to everyone who lacked "means."

"Maurice Mességué, Doctor of Medicine"—that fine brass name plate long shone in my head and in my heart like a ray of hope. I would picture it to myself, and it would dispel all the humiliations the healer had undergone. It would proclaim my right to heal, and for a long time I believed it necessary to my happiness. But then I came to understand that, contrary to what some people might think, mine was the more difficult path: to practice illegally out in the open, to face up to my fellow men and to the courts, to struggle and fight for the right to heal—this was indeed not the easier way.

Who knows, perhaps I wouldn't have made a good doctor? Perhaps I'd have betrayed the long line of Mességués if I'd abandoned their plants in favor of the currently fashionable drugs. Had I not been forced to defend myself, I would not have had to prove the excellence of my methods. I would have made no experiments. I'd have tried nothing new. I am glad to be the one who takes over when the doctors can do no more.

Were I the type to draw up a balance sheet, I'd say that

I have gained more than I've lost: I have been a pioneer of phytotherapy. I believe in the future of phytotherapy, and I am convinced that it will take its rightful future place among the sciences. I am sure that with research it will develop even more, and perhaps one day my name will stand alongside the names of such men as Dr. Pouchet, who in 1897 turned the attention of the medical world once again to the value of herbs. Dr. Pouchet was also the man who gave a scientific name to this branch of knowledge, which has always been classed with "old wives' tales" and "sorcery," by calling it phytotherapy, from the Greek, meaning treatment by plants.

I am certain that we still have a great deal more to learn, and my hope is that one day empiricists will no longer be rejected *a priori,* that they will be granted the right to make known their discoveries, to impart their new-found knowledge to the world, and that the medical profession will be open to all men of integrity.

My father said: "When a stream becomes a river, you don't think about how to stop it but about how to use it."

Appendix I

MY BASIC PREPARATIONS
FOR THE PRINCIPAL CHRONIC DISEASES

I Prescriptions and Methods

To make up these preparations it is first necessary that the dried plants—whether flower, bud, capsule, stem or leaf—should have been crushed with care.

Dried roots are crushed, but roots used semi-fresh should be grated.

Plants that you are recommended to use fresh or semi-fresh, such as broad-leaved plantain, greater celandine, nettle, watercress, cabbage, beet, should be chopped.

Garlic should be crushed.

Warning: Garlic is counter-indicated if you have any kind of dermatosis. Simply omit it from the preparation.

Onion should be grated.

Warning: It is essential to observe the prescribed dosage of greater celandine, corn poppy, buttercup and Roman camomile, otherwise these plants can have an effect contrary to that desired.

Example: Roman camomile, known for its stomachic properties, can actually cause vomiting if the dosage is too large.

Note: with artichoke, only the leaves of the plant should be used, not the edible leaves of the flower.

Buttercup is also known as bitter crowfoot, or *Ranunculus acris.*

Quantities: Are given for a quart of preparation.

Preparation: Boil a quart of water for five minutes. Let it stand. When it is just lukewarm pour it into a container, preferably enamel or plastic. Drop in your mixture of crushed or chopped plants and let macerate for four or five hours, protected from dust. Then pour the preparation into a clean bottle.

Note: Never keep the liquid in a metal container.

This preparation is used for *foot-* and *hand-baths, hip-baths, vaginal douches, poultices, compresses* and *gargles.*

FOOT- AND HAND-BATHS: 1: Boil 2 quarts of water. Let stand for five minutes.

2: Add to the 2 quarts of boiled water ½ pint of plant extracts. The resultant preparation can be kept and re-warmed, but WITH-

OUT BOILING OR ADDING MORE WATER. You can use it for eight days.

3: Take:

> *in the morning before breakfast*:
> a foot-bath for eight minutes as hot as possible.
> *in the evening, before dinner*:
> a hand-bath for eight minutes as hot as possible.

HIP-BATHS: For these you obviously require three or four quarts of basic preparation. The proportions remain the same as for foot- and hand-baths.

VAGINAL DOUCHES: Same proportions as for foot- and hand-baths.

POULTICES: When cabbage, watercress and beet are employed as poultices, the procedure is as follows:

> 1. Chop up a bunch of watercress, or, alternatively, eight to ten leaves of beet or cabbage from which the thick stalk has been removed.
> Beat two egg whites until very stiff.
> Combine the chopped watercress, cabbage or beet with the egg whites.
> Wrap this preparation in coarse muslin, rather than linen, which has too close a weave.
> 2. Coat this poultice with a small liqueur glass of the appropriate basic preparation.
> It is essential that the poultice be applied directly to the skin.

COMPRESSES: Take a piece of flannel folded in four, or a thick wad of medicated cotton-wool, soak it in the preparation and apply directly to the skin.

GARGLES: One liqueur glass of the basic preparation in one pint of boiled water.

II—Dictionary of "Recipes"

In no case discontinue the treatment prescribed by the doctor in charge

ACNE Gastric — Hepatic — Intestinal — Nervous (*see* DERMATOSIS — skin diseases)

AEROPHAGIA (*see* STOMACH)

ALBUMINURIA

> Common Broom (flowers and young shoots)   *two handfuls*
> Onion   *one large grated onion*

Foot- and hand-baths.

> *Note*: The patient suffering from this complaint should keep strictly to the diet prescribed by the doctor in charge.

ALLERGIES
>Garlic   *one crushed head*
>Single seed hawthorn (blossom)   *one handful*
>Greater celandine (flowers and stems, if possible, semi-fresh)
>   *one handful*
>Couch-grass (roots)   *one handful*
>Common broom (flowers)   *one handful*
>Sage (leaves)   *one handful*
>Linden (blossom)   *one handful*

Foot- and hand-baths.

Note: As allergies are very varied in origin, it is only possible to give a general desensitizing treatment.

AMENORRHEA (*see* WOMEN, Diseases of)

ANGINA (*see* THROAT)

ANGINA PECTORIS (*see* HEART)

ANGER-ANXIETY (*see* NERVES)

ARTERIOSCLEROSIS
>Garlic   *two large crushed heads*
>Single seed hawthorn (blossom)   *one handful*
>Greater celandine (leaves and stems semi-fresh if possible) *one
>   handful*
>Common broom (flowers and young shoots)   *one handful*

Foot- and hand-baths.

Note: For this disease a diet recommended by the doctor should be followed.

ARTERITIS   Inflammation of the arteries
>Garlic   *one large crushed head*
>Artichoke (leaves)   *one handful*
>Single seed hawthorn (blossom)   *one handful*
>Sage (flowers and leaves)   *one handful*
>Thyme (leaves and flowers)   *one handful*

Foot- and hand-baths.

Note: As arteritis may stem from a variety of causes, the basic treatment can only alleviate but cannot cure.

ARTHRITIS
>Garlic   *one large crushed head*
>Greater celandine (leaves, semi-fresh if possible)   *one handful*
>Nettle (leaves and stems, semi-fresh if possible)   *two handfuls*
>Dandelion (whole plant, semi-fresh if possible)   *one handful*
>Meadow-sweet (flowers)   *one handful*
>Buttercup (flowers and leaves)   *one handful*

Foot- and hand-baths.

Note: While no special diet need be followed, certain foods and drinks are inadvisable.

ASTHMA

Garlic   *one large crushed head*
Corn poppy (flowers and capsules)   *one handful*
Lavender (flowers)   *one handful*
Ground-ivy (leaves)   *one handful*
Parsley (leaves)   *one handful*
Sage (flowers)   *one handful*
Thyme (flowers)   *one handful*

Foot- and hand-baths.

Note: Since asthma stems from a variety of allergies, the patient should follow the doctor's treatment suited to his own case. This preparation can only bring relief during an attack and is not a cure.

BLADDER (Diseases of the)

CYSTITIS:

Spring heath (flowers)   *one handful*
Corn poppy (flowers and crushed capsules)   *one handful*
Corn (stigma)   *one handful*
Round-leaved mallow (grated root)   *one handful*
Broad-leaved plantain (leaves, fresh if possible)   *one handful*

Hip-baths. Vaginal douches.

Note: For this condition it is advisable to take dietary precautions, as recommended by the doctor, and particularly to cut out certain foods and drinks.

INCONTINENCE OF URINE

Garlic   *one large crushed head*
Single seed hawthorn (blossom)   *one handful*
Buttercup (leaves and flowers)   *one handful*

Hip-baths.

PROSTATE:

Single seed hawthorn (blossom)   *one handful*
Borage (flowers)   *one handful*
Spring heath (flowers)   *half handful*
Greater celandine (leaves, fresh if possible)   *one handful*
Round-leaved mallow (grated root)   *one handful*

Hip-baths.

BOWELS (Functional disorders of the)

Note: In these cases it is advisable to follow the diet prescribed by the doctor.

CONSTIPATION:

Artichoke (leaves)   *one handful*
Roman camomile   *one dozen crushed heads*
Succory, or chicory (leaves and roots)   *one handful*
Cabbage (leaves)   *one handful*
Bindweed (flowers and leaves)   *one handful*
Round-leaved mallow (flowers)   *one handful*
Onion   *one large grated onion*
Thyme (flowers)   *one handful*
Sweet violet (flowers)   *one handful*

Foot- and hand-baths.

Lavender (flowers)   *one handful*
Ground-ivy (leaves)   *one handful*
Parsley (leaves)   *one handful*
Sage (flowers)   *one handful*
Thyme (flowers)   *one handful*

Foot- and hand-baths.

ENTERITIS (DYSENTERY):

Round-leaved mallow (flowers and roots)   *one handful*
Nettle (leaves, fresh if possible)   *one handful*
Knot-grass (whole plant)   *one handful*
Field horsetail (stems and young shoots)   *one handful*

Foot- and hand-baths.

BRONCHIAL DISEASES

Basic preparation:
Garlic   *one large crushed head*
Borage (flowers and leaves)   *one handful*
Cabbage (fresh leaves)   *one handful*
or
Corn poppy (flowers and capsules)   *one handful*
Watercress (fresh leaves)   *one bunch*
Sage (flowers)   *one handful*
Sweet violet (flowers)   *one handful*

BRONCHITIS, CHRONIC

Corn poppy (flowers and capsules)   *one handful*
Lavender (flowers)   *one handful*
Ground-ivy (leaves)   *one handful*
Round-leaved mallow (flowers)   *one handful*
Onion   *one large grated*
Sage (flowers and leaves)   *one handful*

Foot- and hand-baths.

BUZZING IN THE EARS

>Single seed hawthorn (blossom)   *one handful*
>Buttercup (flowers and leaves)   *one handful*
>Dandelion (whole plant, semi-fresh if possible)   *one handful*
>Sage (flowers and leaves)   *one handful*

Foot- and hand-baths.

CALCULI (*see* LITHIASIS, URINARY)

CATARRH, BRONCHIAL AND PULMONARY (*see* BRONCHIAL diseases)
Same treatment as for bronchial complaints. Increase the dose of round-leaved mallow or sweet violet: two handfuls instead of one.

CELLULITIS

>Spring heath (flowers)   *one handful*
>Sour Cherries (stems)   *one handful*
>Greater celandine (stems and flowers, semi-fresh if possible)   *one handful*
>Couch-grass (roots)   *one handful*
>Common broom (flowers and young shoots)   *one handful*
>Corn (stigma)   *one handful*
>Onion   *one large grated*
>Field horsetail (leaves)   *one handful*
>Meadow-sweet (flowers)   *one handful*

Foot- and hand-baths.

If you are unable to obtain all these plants, an excellent diuretic can be made from:

>Greater celandine (stems and flowers, semi-fresh if possible)   *one handful*
>Corn (stigma)   *two handfuls*
>Meadow-sweet (flowers)   *one handful*
>Field horsetail (leaves)   *one handful*

Foot- and hand-baths.

>*Note*: This basic treatment will be effective only if accompanied by a controlled diet suggested by the doctor.

CHOLECYSTITIS (*see* LITHIASIS, BILIARY - LIVER)

CHOLESTEROL (Excess of) (*see* LIVER)

CIRRHOSIS OF THE LIVER (*see* LIVER)

COLIC, HEPATIC (*see* LITHIASIS, BILIARY - LIVER)

COLIC, NEPHRITIC

>Buttercup (flowers and leaves)   *one handful*
>Couch-grass (roots)   *one handful*
>Corn (stigma)   *one handful*
>Round-leaved mallow (flowers)   *one handful*

Hip-baths.

Note: Nephritic or renal colic is the painful sign of urinary lithiasis. This basic preparation is intended to relieve the pain. For treatment of the causes, *see* Lithiasis, Urinary.

COLLIBACILLOSIS

 Buttercup (flowers and leaves) *one handful*
 Spring heath (flowers) *one handful*
 Round-leaved mallow (flowers) *one handful*
 Broad-leaved plantain (leaves) *one handful*
 Sage (flowers and leaves) *one handful*

Hip-baths.

Note: Some care should be taken over diet, and certain foods and drinks should be avoided, as suggested by your doctor.

CONSTIPATION (*see* BOWELS)

COUGH

 Borage (leaves and stems) *one handful*
 Corn poppy (flowers and crushed capsules) *one handful*
 Ground-ivy (stems and leaves) *one handful*
 Round-leaved mallow (grated roots) *one handful*
 Peppermint (flowers and leaves) *one handful*
 Parsley (chopped, fresh if possible) *one handful*
 Sweet violet (flowers) *one handful*

Foot- and hand-baths.

CYSTITIS (*see* BLADDER)

DEPRESSION, NERVOUS (*see* NERVES)

DERMATOSIS

Note: Acne can be due to different causes—liver, bowels, stomach, change of life—and the basic treatment will only bring relief but not cure the condition. For all skin diseases it is important to follow the diet prescribed by the doctor.

ACNE:

 Great burdock (flowers and leaves) *one handful*
 Marshmallow (chopped root) *one handful*
 Round-leaved mallow (flowers) *one handful*
 Onion *one large grated*
 Sage (flowers and leaves) *one handful*

Hot compresses to be applied locally, and foot- and hand-baths.

Note: This preparation, to the exclusion of all others, can be used on acne rash.

In cases when the origin of the acne has been determined by the doctor in charge, I recommend the following treatments:

ACNE OF HEPATIC ORIGIN:

> *Basic preparation:*
> Artichoke (leaves)   *one handful*
> Great burdock (leaves)   *one handful*
> Greater celandine (leaves, fresh if possible)   *one handful*
> Round-leaved mallow (flowers and roots)   *one handful*
> Sage (flowers)   *one handful*
> *Poultice:* cabbage and onion

Coat the poultice with a small liqueur glass of the basic preparation and apply over the liver.

Foot- and hand-baths with basic preparation only.

ACNE OF GASTRIC ORIGIN:

> Garlic   *one large crushed head*
> Great burdock (leaves)   *one handful*
> Roman camomile   *one dozen crushed heads*
> Greater celandine (leaves, semi-fresh if possible)   *one handful*
> Peppermint (leaves)   *one handful*
> Nettle (leaves, fresh if possible)   *one handful*
> Thyme (leaves)   *one handful*

Poultice: Cabbage and watercress, coated with a small liqueur glass of basic preparation, applied to stomach.

Foot- and hand-baths with basic preparation only.

ACNE OF INTESTINAL ORIGIN:

> Garlic   *one large crushed head*
> Great burdock (flowers and leaves)   *one handful*
> Roman camomile   *one dozen crushed heads*
> Greater celandine (leaves and flowers, semi-fresh if possible)
>   *one handful*
> Field bindweed (flowers)   *one handful*
> Round-leaved mallow (flowers)   *one handful*

Poultice: Cabbage (fresh leaves) and nettle (leaves, fresh if possible), to be coated with a liqueur glass of basic preparation and applied to the stomach.

Foot- and hand-baths with basic preparation only.

ACNE OF NERVOUS ORIGIN:

> Single seed hawthorn (blossom)   *one handful*
> Greater celandine (leaves, semi-fresh if possible)   *one handful*
> Corn poppy (flowers and capsules)   *one handful*
> Sweet brier (petals and buds)   *one handful*
> Nettle (leaves, fresh if possible)   *one handful*
> Linden (blossom)   *one handful*

Foot- and hand-baths.

SKIN TROUBLE

ECZEMA

ERYSIPELAS

The various causes should be treated individually, but excellent results are obtained with the following general treatment:

Artichoke (leaves)   *one handful*
Elecampane (flowers and leaves)   *one handful*
Great burdock (leaves)   *one handful*
Buttercup (flowers and leaves)   *one handful*
Greater celandine (leaves, semi-fresh if possible)   *one handful*
Succory, or chicory (roots and tips)   *one handful*
Common broom (flowers)   *one handful*
Lavender (flowers)   *one handful*
Nettle (leaves, fresh if possible)   *one handful*

Foot- and hand-baths.

ITCHING or PRURITUS

Elecampane (flowers)   *one handful*
Great burdock (flowers and leaves)   *one handful*
Marsh-mallow (chopped root)   *one handful*
Dandelion (grated root)   *one handful*
Broad-leaved plantain (leaves, fresh if possible)   *one handful*
Cabbage rose (petals)   *one handful*

Foot- and hand-baths. Local applications: See that it penetrates the skin but do not rub. Hip-baths, if necessary, to which a handful of starch has been added.

FURUNCULOSIS

Treatment as for acne, it having the same origins.

Note: To the basic preparation add onion (one large grated), a handful of broad-leaved plantain (fresh leaves), a handful of marsh-mallow (chopped root), and double the quantity of round-leaved mallow.

Compress to be applied to the boils.

Foot- and hand-baths.

HERPES:

Borage (flowers)   *one handful*
Greater celandine (leaves, semi-fresh, if possible)   *one handful*
Corn poppy (flowers and crushed capsules)   *half handful*
Marsh-mallow (chopped root)   *one handful*
Round-leaved mallow (flowers and roots)   *one handful*

Hip-baths if appropriate.

Vaginal douche.

Foot- and hand-baths.

Warning: Do not use this preparation as a mouthwash.

IMPETIGO:

>   Great burdock (flowers and leaves)   *one handful*
>   Corn poppy (flowers and crushed capsules)   *one handful*
>   Broad-leaved plantain (leaves and flowers)   *one handful*
>   Sage (leaves and flowers)   *one handful*

Apply lightly to affected areas.

Foot- and hand-baths.

URTICARIA:

>   Greater celandine (flowers and stems, semi-fresh if possible)
>   *one handful*
>   Corn poppy (flowers and crushed capsules)   *one handful*
>   Round-leaved mallow (flowers and leaves)   *one handful*
>   Nettle (leaves, fresh if possible)   *one handful*
>   Sage (flowers and leaves)   *one handful*
>   Sweet violet (flowers)   *one handful*

Apply locally without rubbing.

Foot- and hand-baths.

SHINGLES:

>   Buttercup (flowers and leaves)   *one handful*
>   Corn poppy (flowers and crushed capsules)   *one handful*
>   Meadow-sweet (flowers)   *one handful*
>   Linden (blossom)   *one handful*

Local compresses.

Foot- and hand-baths.

In the case of eruption all over the body, a linden-blossom bath is to be recommended: 17½ ounces to a quart of water. Its soothing action can be increased by a handful of corn poppy and made milder by two handfuls of round-leaved mallow (flowers or root) and three handfuls of starch.

DIGESTION (Disturbances of) (*see* STOMACH)

DIZZINESS

>   Single seed hawthorn (blossom)   *one handful*
>   Roman camomile   *one dozen crushed heads*
>   Lavender (flowers)   *one handful*
>   Peppermint (flowers and leaves)   *one handful*
>   Sage (flowers and leaves)   *one handful*

Foot- and hand-baths.

DROPSY

>   Greater celandine (leaves, semi-fresh if possible)   *one handful*
>   Watercress   *one bunch*
>   Common broom (flowers)   *one handful*
>   Onion   *one large grated*

Parsley (fresh leaves) *one handful*
Field horsetail (stems and young shoots) *one handful*
or
Meadow-sweet (flowers) *one handful*
  Foot- and hand-baths.

DYSMENORRHEA (*see* WOMEN, Diseases of)
DYSPEPSIA (*see* STOMACH)
ECZEMA (*see* DERMATOSIS)
EMOTIVITY (*see* NERVES)

EMPHYSEMA

Garlic *one large crushed head*
Single seed hawthorn (blossom) *one handful*
Ground-ivy (leaves) *one handful*
Sage (flowers and leaves) *one handful*
Thyme (leaves) *one handful*
  Foot- and hand-baths.

ENTERITIS or DYSENTERY (*see* BOWELS)
ERYSIPELAS (*see* DERMATOSIS)
FLATULENCE and WIND (*see* BOWELS)
FRIGIDITY (*see* WOMEN, DISEASES OF)
FURUNCULOSIS (*see* DERMATOSIS)
GASTRALGIA (*see* STOMACH)
GASTRITIS (*see* STOMACH)
GOUT

Note: For this illness the patient should adhere to a very strict
diet, as prescribed by the doctor.
Great burdock (stems, leaves) *one handful*
Roman camomile *one dozen crushed heads*
Couch-grass (grated roots) *one handful*
Cabbage (leaves) *one handful*
Autumn crocus (can be used alone) *one handful*
Male fern (grated roots) *one handful*
Common broom (flowers) *one handful*
Lavender (flowers) *one handful*
Sage (flowers and leaves) *one handful*
  Foot- and hand-baths.

HEMORRHOIDS

Note: For this treatment to have maximum effect, it is advisable
to follow a diet, as prescribed by the doctor.
Milfoil (flowers) *one handful*
Milk-thistle (roots and leaves) *one handful*
Couch-grass (grated roots) *one handful*
Lavender (flowers) *one handful*

Field horsetail (plants)   *one handful*
Knot-grass (grated roots)   *one handful*
Hip-baths.

HEART (Functional disturbances of)

ANGINA PECTORIS and INFARCTUS:

Single seed hawthorn (blossom)   *one handful*
Buttercup (stems and leaves)   *one handful*
Greater celandine (stems and leaves, semi-fresh if possible) *one handful*
Common broom (flowers and young shoots)   *one handful*

Attacks: Compress over the heart, to be kept on all night.
Regular treatment: Foot- and hand-baths.

EDEMA OF THE HEART:

Single seed hawthorn (blossom)   *one handful*
Greater celandine (leaves and stems, fresh if possible) *one handful*
Common broom (leaves and young shoots)   *one handful*
Onion   *one large grated*
Meadow-sweet (flowers)   *one handful*

Attacks: Compress on the heart.
Regular treatment: Hand-baths.

PALPITATIONS:

Single seed hawthorn (blossom)   *one handful*
Buttercup (flowers and leaves)   *one handful*
Sweet brier (petals and crushed buds)   *one handful*
Peppermint (leaves)   *one handful*
Sage (leaves)   *one handful*

Attacks: Compress over the heart.
Regular treatment: Foot- and hand-baths.

PERICARDITIS:

Single seed hawthorn (blossom and buds)   *one handful*
Onion   *one large grated*
Sage (leaves)   *one handful*

Foot- and hand-baths.

TACHYCARDIA:

Single seed hawthorn (blossom and buds)   *one handful*
Buttercup (flowers and leaves)   *one handful*
Milk-thistle (roots and leaves)   *one handful*
Sweet brier (petals and buds)   *one handful*

Attacks: Compress over the heart.
Regular treatment: Foot- and hand-baths.

Note: In certain of these conditions it is advisable to eliminate all stimulants from the diet.

HERPES (*see* DERMATOSIS)

HOARSENESS (*see* THROAT)

HYPERACIDITY (*see* STOMACH)

HYPERTENSION

Note: It is advisable to follow the diet prescribed by the doctor in charge.

Garlic   *one large crushed head*
Single seed hawthorn (blossom)   *one handful*
Greater celandine (leaves, semi-fresh if possible)   *one handful*
Common broom (flowers)   *one handful*

Foot- and hand-baths.

ICTERUS — CHRONIC JAUNDICE (*see* LIVER)

IMPETIGO (*see* DERMATOSIS)

IMPOTENCE

Cow-parsley (roots, leaves, seed)   *four pinches*
Buttercup (leaves and flowers)   *one handful*
Greater celandine (leaves, semi-fresh if possible)   *one handful*
Fenugreek (crushed seeds)   *one and a half handfuls*
Peppermint (leaves)   *one handful*
Summer savory (leaves)   *one handful*

Hip-baths.

INCONTINENCE OF URINE (*see* BLADDER)

INFARCTUS AND ANGINA PECTORIS (*see* HEART)

INSOMNIA

Note: Linden-blossom baths give excellent results (1 4/5 oz. of linden blossoms to one quart of water). They render unnecessary any chemical sleeping-pill or sedative, and are particularly recommended for infants and children.

Persons using linden blossom for infusions are warned to make them mild, for a strong dose of linden blossom will cause insomnia.

Single seed hawthorn (blossom)   *one handful*
Corn poppy (flowers and crushed capsules)   *one handful*
Peppermint (leaves)   *one handful*
Linden (blossom)   *one handful*

Foot- and hand-baths.

ITCHING (*see* DERMATOSIS)

JAUNDICE, CHRONIC OR ICTERUS (*see* LIVER)

LARYNGITIS (*see* THROAT)

LEUKORRHEA, OR WHITES (*see* WOMEN, DISEASES OF)

LITHIASIS, BILIARY (*see* LIVER)

LITHIASIS, URNINARY (or CALCULI)

Note: For this condition it is advisable to follow the diet prescribed by the doctor.

Great burdock (flowers, leaves)   *one handful*
Borage (flowers)   *one handful*
Greater celandine (leaves, semi-fresh if possible)   *one handful*
Couch-grass (grated roots)   *one handful*
Sweet brier (fruit, petals, buds)   *one handful*
Common broom (flowers)   *one handful*
Corn (stigma)   *one handful*

Compresses to be applied over the kidneys.
Foot- and hand-baths.

LIVER (Diseases of the)

Note: Since diseases or functional disorders of the liver stem from different causes (liver or gall bladder), this preparation does not treat the cause but only the effect: attacks of pain, digestive troubles, nausea. It may be considered as an excellent basic and general treatment. For all diseases of the liver it is important to follow a suitable diet, prescribed by the doctor.

Milfoil (flowers)   *one handful*
Garlic   *one crushed head*
Artichoke (leaves)   *one handful*
Greater celandine (leaves and stems, semi-fresh if possible)   *one handful*
Succory, or chicory (grated roots)   *one handful*
Couch-grass (grated roots)   *one handful*
Hedge-bindweed (Rutland Beauty) (flowers and leaves)   *one handful*
Sage (leaves)   *one handful*

Poultice: Cabbage and kale, coated with a liqueur glass of the basic preparation.
Treatment: Foot- and hand-baths with basic preparation only.

ICTERUS OR CHRONIC JAUNDICE:

Artichoke (leaves)   *one handful*
Greater celandine (leaves and stems)   *one handful*
mixed } Succory, or chicory (leaves)
Dandelion (whole plant)   *one handful*
Couch-grass (grated roots)   *one handful*
Foot- and hand-baths.

HEPATIC INSUFFICIENCY:

Artichoke (leaves)   *one handful*
Greater celandine (leaves and stems, semi-fresh if possible)   *one handful*

Succory, chicory (leaves) ⎫
Dandelion (whole plants) ⎬ *one handful*
Hedge-bindweed (Rutland Beauty) (flowers and leaves)
    one handful

Foot- and hand-baths.

CHOLESTEROL (Excess of)
    Artichoke (leaves)   *one handful*
    Single seed hawthorn (blossom)   *one handful*
    Milk-thistle (roots and leaves)   *one handful*
    Greater celandine (flowers and stems)   *one handful*
    Couch-grass (leaves)   *one handful*

Foot- and hand-baths.

CIRRHOSIS OF THE LIVER
    Artichoke (leaves)   *one handful*
    Greater celandine (flowers and stems)   *one handful*
    Cabbage (leaves)   *one handful*

Compresses applied over the liver.

Foot- and hand-baths.

BILIARY LITHIASIS OR HEPATIC COLIC (Calculi)
    Note: This treatment is not a substitute for surgery when the
    latter is necessary. It merely facilitates the passage of sediment.
    Artichoke (leaves)   *one handful*

mixed ⎰ Succory, or chicory (leaves and roots) ⎱ *one handful*
       ⎱ Dandelion (leaves and roots) ⎰
    Couch-grass (grated roots)   *one handful*
    Corn poppy (petals and capsules)   *one handful*

Hot compresses to be applied over the gall bladder.
Foot- and hand-baths.

LOW BLOOD PRESSURE
    Note: It is advisable to follow the diet prescribed by the doctor
    in charge.
    Single seed hawthorn (blossom)   *one handful*
    Cow-parsnip (roots, leaves)   *one handful*
    Milk-thistle (roots, leaves)   *one handful*
    Corn (stigma)   *one handful*

Foot- and hand-baths.

LUMBAGO (*see* NERVES)

LUNG (*see* BRONCHIAL DISEASES)

MENOPAUSE (*see* WOMEN, DISEASES OF)

METRORRHAGIA (*see* WOMEN, DISEASES OF)

MIGRAINE

Note: The causes of migraine are varied. The basic preparation will relieve the symptoms but does not treat the cause.

Roman camomile *five crushed heads*
Lavender (flowers) *one handful*
Melissa or citronella (leaves) *one handful*
Officinal primula (leaves and flowers, roots if possible) *one handful*

Acute attack: Iced compresses on the forehead.

Regular treatment: Foot- and hand-baths.

MIGRAINE IN WOMEN:

Greater celandine (leaves, semi-fresh) *one handful*
Melissa or citronella (leaves) *one handful*
Peppermint (leaves and flowers) *one handful*
Parsley (fresh leaves) *one handful*

Acute attack: Iced compresses on the forehead.

Foot- and hand-baths.

Follow the treatment for the woman's illness in question.

MIGRAINE OF HEPATIC ORIGIN:

Artichoke (leaves, fresh if possible) *one handful*
Greater celandine (leaves, semi-fresh) *one handful*
Melissa or citronella (leaves) *one handful*
Peppermint (leaves and flowers) *one handful*

Acute attack: Iced compresses on the forehead. Follow the appropriate liver treatment prescribed by the doctor.

MIGRAINE OF INTESTINAL ORIGIN:

Roman camomile *one dozen crushed heads*
Greater celandine (leaves, semi-fresh if possible) *one handful*
Melissa or citronella (leaves) *one handful*
Bindweed (flowers and leaves) *one handful*
Peppermint (leaves and flowers) *one handful*

Acute attack: Iced compresses on the forehead.

Regular treatment: Foot- and hand-baths as prescribed for constipation.

MIGRAINE OF NERVOUS ORIGIN:

Single seed hawthorn (blossom and buds) *one handful*
Roman camomile *one dozen crushed heads*
Peppermint (leaves and flowers) *one handful*
Officinal primula (leaves and flowers, roots if possible) *one handful*
Sweet violet (flowers) *one handful*

Acute attack: Iced compresses on the forehead.

Regular treatment: Foot- and hand-baths as prescribed for nerves.

MIGRAINE OF OPHTHALMIC ORIGIN:

Roman camomile   *one dozen crushed heads*
Greater celandine (leaves, semi-fresh if possible)   *one handful*
Round-leaved mallow (grated roots)   *one handful*
Broad-leaved plantain (leaves)   *one handful*
Cabbage rose (petals)   *one handful*
Sweet violet (flowers)   *one handful*

Compresses on the eyes. Proportions: a small liqueur glass to one-half pint of boiled water.

Note: For eye compresses, discard the liquid once it has been used.

NERVES

Basic regular treatment:
Single seed hawthorn (blossom)   *one handful*
Sweet brier (petals and buds)   *one handful*
Peppermint (leaves and flowers)   *one handful*
Sage (leaves)   *one handful*

Foot- and hand-baths.

Note: An excellent sedative for the nerves in general is a linden-blossom bath: 500g of blossoms to a quart of water.

ANGER-ANXIETY:

Single seed hawthorn (blossom)   *one handful*
Corn poppy (flowers and capsules)   *one handful*
Sweet brier (petals and buds)   *one handful*
Meadow-sweet (flowers)   *one handful*

Foot- and hand-baths.

NERVOUS DEPRESSION:

Single seed hawthorn (blossom)   *one handful*
Sage (leaves and flowers)   *one handful*
Sweet violet (flowers)   *one handful*

Foot- and hand-baths.

EMOTIVITY:

Single seed hawthorn (blossom)   *one handful*
Knapweed (leaves)   *one handful*
Meadow-sweet (flowers)   *one handful*
Linden (blossom)   *half handful*

Foot- and hand-baths.

DISORDERS OF THE SYMPATHETIC NERVOUS SYSTEM:

Basic preparation as for Nerves, with the addition of a handful of corn poppy (flowers and crushed capsules) and buttercup (leaves and flowers).

Foot- and hand-baths.

STATE OF NERVES, IRRITABILITY

Note: As this condition can stem from different causes, the following basic treatment is merely sedative in effect and cannot treat the cause.

Single seed hawthorn (blossom)   *one handful*
Greater celandine (leaves, semi-fresh if possible)   *one handful*
Corn poppy (flowers and crushed capsules)   *one handful*
Peppermint (leaves and flowers)   *one handful*
Sage (leaves and flowers)   *one handful*

Foot- and hand-baths.

NEURALGIA

Roman camomile   *one dozen crushed heads*
Corn poppy (flowers and crushed capsules)   *one handful*
Peppermint (flowers and leaves)   *one handful*
Meadow-sweet (flowers)   *one handful*

Note: For very acute cases of neuralgia add a handful of buttercup.

LUMBAGO:

Single seed hawthorn (blossom)   *one handful*
Great burdock (flowers and leaves)   *one handful*
Buttercup (leaves and flowers)   *one handful*
Onion   *one large grated*
Nettle (leaves, fresh if possible)   *one handful*

Compresses over the kidneys.

Foot- and hand-baths.

FACIAL NEURALGIA:

Buttercup (leaves and flowers)   *one handful*
Greater celandine (leaves, semi-fresh if possible)   *one handful*
Cabbage (leaves)   *one handful*
Thyme (flowers)   *one handful*

Foot- and hand-baths.

PALPITATIONS (*see* HEART)
PERICARDITIS (*see* HEART)
PERIODS (*see* WOMEN, DISEASES OF)
PHARYNGITIS (*see* THROAT)
PROSTATE (*see* BLADDER)
PRURITIS (ITCHING, *see* DERMATOSIS)
RHEUMATISM

Note: In the event of an acute attack of rheumatism, pain will be speedily alleviated by using a maceration of buttercup flowers and leaves: six handfuls to a quart of water. This preparation will rid the patient of pain, but it does not treat the causes of the pain.

Follow it up with this basic treatment:

Great burdock (leaves)   *one handful*
Spring heath (flowers)   *one handful*
Roman camomile   *one dozen crushed heads*
Greater celandine (leaves and stems, semi-fresh if possible)
   one handful
Couch-grass (grated roots)   *one handful*
Common broom (flowers)   *one handful*
Lavender (flowers)   *one handful*
Onion   *one large grated*

Poultices: Cabbage, watercress or kale, coated with a liqueur glass of the basic preparation.

Poultices are to be applied only in the event of acute attack and to the affected areas, directly to the skin. They do not replace hand- and foot-baths, which are the curative treatment.

SCIATICA

Buttercup (leaves and flowers)   *one handful*
Greater celandine (leaves, fresh if possible)   *one handful*
Cabbage (leaves)   *one handful*
Peppermint (flowers and leaves)   *one handful*
Thyme (flowers)   *one handful*

Hip-baths.

Foot- and hand-baths.

SHINGLES (*see* DERMATOSIS)

SKIN (Diseases of the) (*see* DERMATOSIS)

SKIN TROUBLE (*see* DERMATOSIS)

SPASMS, GASTRIC (*see* STOMACH)

STERILITY (*see* WOMEN, DISEASES OF)

STOMACH (Complaints of the)

Note: As functional disorders of the digestive tract may have different causes—hepatic, psychosomatic, etc.—these basic treatments should be followed only when the causes have been determined by the doctor in charge. For all stomach disorders the patient should follow the diet prescribed for his case by the doctor.

AEROPHAGIA:

Milfoil (flowers)   *one handful*
Single seed hawthorn (blossom)   *one handful*
Elecampane (flowers)   *one handful*
Buttercup (flowers and leaves)   *one handful*
Peppermint (leaves)   *one handful*
Blackberry bramble (leaves)   *one handful*
Sage (leaves and flowers)   *one handful*

Hot compresses to be applied to the stomach, preferably immediately after meals.

Hand-baths.

DIGESTION (Disorders of the)

>*Basic Preparation:*
>Garlic   *one large crushed head*
>Roman camomile   *one dozen crushed heads*
>Peppermint (leaves)   *one handful*
>Thyme (leaves)   *one handful*

Poultices: Nettle (fresh leaves if possible), watercress (one bunch, chopped). Add a liqueur glass of basic preparation. To be applied hot, after meals.

Hand-baths with basic preparation only.

DYSPEPSIA:

>Milfoil (flowers)   *one handful*
>Garlic   *one large crushed head*
>Cow-parsnip (root, leaves, seed)   *one handful, mixed*
>Roman camomile   *one dozen crushed heads*
>or
>Peppermint (leaves)   *one handful*
>Yellow gentian (root)   *one large pinch*
>Round-leaved mallow (leaves and flowers)   *one handful*
>Thyme (leaves)   *one handful*

Foot- and hand-baths.

GASTRALGIA:

>Milfoil (flowers)   *one handful*
>Garlic   *one crushed head*
>Single seed hawthorn (blossom)   *one handful*
>Corn poppy (flowers and capsules)   *one handful*
>Round-leaved mallow (flowers and leaves)   *one handful*
>Blackberry bramble (leaves)   *one handful*

Hot compresses to be applied to the stomach.

Hand-baths.

GASTRITIS:

>Roman camomile   *one dozen crushed heads*
>Greater celandine (leaves and stems, semi-fresh if possible)   *one handful*
>Corn poppy (flowers and crushed capsules)   *one handful*
>Round-leaved mallow (leaves and stems)   *one handful*
>Nettle (leaves, fresh if possible)   *one handful*

Lukewarm compresses to be applied to the stomach.

Hand-baths.

HYPERACIDITY:

> Single seed hawthorn (blossom)   *one handful*
> Sweet brier (crushed seeds)   *one handful*
> Lavender (flowers)   *one handful*
> Round-leaved mallow (flowers and leaves)   *one handful*
> Peppermint (leaves)   *one handful*

Foot- and hand-baths.

GASTRIC SPASMS:

> Single seed hawthorn (blossom)   *one handful*
> Sweet brier (crushed seeds)   *one handful*
> Roman camomile (flowers)   *one dozen crushed heads*
> Greater celandine (leaves and stems, semi-fresh if possible) *one handful*
> Corn poppy (flowers and crushed capsules)   *one handful*
> Lavender (flowers)   *one handful*
> Peppermint (leaves and flowers)   *one handful*

Hot compresses to be applied to the stomach.

Hand-baths.

ULCERS (of the STOMACH and the DUODENUM)

> Single seed hawthorn (blossom)   *one handful*
> Greater celandine (flowers and stems, semi-fresh if possible) *one handful*
> Couch-grass (leaves)   *one handful*
> Corn poppy (flowers and capsules)   *one handful*
> Blackberry bramble (leaves)   *one handful*
> Sage (leaves and flowers)   *one handful*
> Sweet violet (flowers)   *one handful*

Poultice: Fresh cabbage (leaves), watercress (one bunch), nettle (leaves), fresh if possible.

During an attack: Hot poultice. Add a liqueur glass of basic preparation.

Treatment: Hand- and foot-baths with basic preparation only.

SYMPATHETIC NERVOUS SYSTEM (disorders of the) (*see* NERVES)

TACHYCARDIA (*see* HEART)

THROAT (complaints)

> *Note*: Throat diseases can arise from varied causes: growths, tonsils, various infections. This preparation should therefore be considered only as basic treatment.

> Single seed hawthorn (blossom)   *one handful*
> Corn poppy (flowers and crushed capsules)   *one handful*
> Round-leaved mallow (grated roots)   *one handful*
> Blackberry brambles (leaves)   *one handful*
> Cabbage rose (petals)   *one handful*

Field horsetail (stems)   *one handful*
Sweet violet (flowers)   *one handful*

Used as gargle or throat-wash. Proportions: One liqueur glass to ½ pint of boiled water.

ANGINA:

Nettle (leaves, fresh if possible)   *one handful*
Broad-leaved plantain (leaves)   *one handful*
Cabbage rose (petals)   *one handful*
Sweet violet (flowers)   *one handful*

Used as gargle or throat-wash. Proportions: One small liqueur glass to ½ pint of boiled water.

TONSILLITIS:

Nettle (leaves, fresh if possible)   *one handful*
Broad-leaved plantain (leaves)   *one handful*
Blackberry brambles (leaves)   *one handful*
Cabbage rose (petals)   *one handful*
Sage (flowers)   *one handful*
Sweet violet (flowers)   *one handful*

Used as gargle or throat-wash. Proportions: One small liqueur glass to ½ pint of boiled water.

PHARYNGITIS:

Single seed hawthorn (blossom)   *one handful*
Round-leaved mallow (flowers)   *one handful*
Blackberry brambles (leaves)   *one handful*
Sweet violet (flowers)   *one handful*

Used as gargle or throat-wash. Proportions: One small liqueur glass to ½ pint of boiled water.

HOARSENESS:

LARYNGITIS:

Cabbage (leaves)   *one handful*
Lavender (flowers)   *one handful*
Round-leaved mallow (flowers)   *one handful*
Broad-leaved plantain (leaves)   *one handful*
Sweet violet (flowers)   *one handful*

Used as gargle or throat-wash. Proportions: One small liqueur glass to ½ pint of boiled water.

TRACHEITIS:

Elecampane (flowers)   *one handful*
Couch-grass (roots)   *one handful*
Cabbage (leaves)   *one handful*
Corn poppy (flowers)   *one handful*
Round-leaved mallow (flowers)   *one handful*
Sweet violet (flowers)   *one handful*

Used as gargle or throat-wash. Proportions: One small liqueur glass to ½ pint of boiled water.

Note: This preparation is excellent for all smokers.

TRACHEITIS (*see* THROAT)

TORTICOLLIS (Stiff neck)

 Onion *one large grated*

 Rosemary (leaves) *one handful*

 Thyme (flowers) *one handful*

Local compresses.

TRACHEITIS (*see* THROAT)

ULCERS (Duodenal, Stomach) (*see* STOMACH)

ULCERS, VARICOSE

 Great burdock (roots and leaves) *one handful*

 Knapweed (leaves) *one handful*

 Ground-ivy (leaves) *one handful*

 Broad-leaved plantain or red rose (leaves) *one handful*

 Blackberry brambles (leaves) *one handful*

 Sage (flowers and leaves) *one handful*

Hand-baths.

Note: Warning — no foot-baths for varicose veins.

UREMIA

 Note: It is advisable to follow a diet prescribed by the doctor.

 Greater celandine (leaves and stems, semi-fresh if possible) *one handful*

 Common broom (flowers) *one handful*

 Meadow-sweet (flowers) *one handful*

Foot- and hand-baths.

URTICARIA (*see* DERMATOSIS)

VAGINITIS (*see* WOMEN, DISEASES OF)

VARICOSE VEINS

 Single seed hawthorn (blossom) *one handful*

 Milfoil (flowers) *one handful*

 Common broom (flowers) *one handful*

 Meadow-sweet (flowers) *one handful*

Foot- and hand-baths.

WOMEN (Diseases of)

AMENORRHEA:

 Milfoil (flowers) *one handful*

 Elecampane (flowers) *one handful*

 Parsley (fresh if possible) *one handful*

 Field-horsetail (leaves) *two handfuls*

 Sage (flowers and leaves) *one handful*

Vaginal douches.

DYSMENORRHEA:
>   Milfoil (flowers)   *one handful*
>   Peppermint (leaves, fresh)   *one handful*
>   Parsley (fresh if possible)   *one handful*
>   Sage (flowers and leaves)   *one handful*

Vaginal douches.

FRIGIDITY:
>   Cow-parsnip (root)   *one handful*
>   Greater celandine (leaves and stems, semi-fresh if possible)
>   *one handful*
>   Fenugreek (crushed seeds)   *½ oz.*
>   Peppermint (leaves)   *one handful*
>   Broad-leaved plantain (leaves, fresh if possible, chopped)
>   *one handful*
>   Summer savory (leaves)   *one handful*

Vaginal douches.

LEUKORRHEA, OR WHITES:
>   Elecampane (leaves)   *one handful*
>   Buttercup (leaves and flowers)   *one handful*
>   Knot-grass (crushed roots)   *one handful*
>   Blackberry brambles (leaves)   *one handful*
>   Cabbage roses (petals)   *one handful*
>   Sage (leaves)   *one handful*

Vaginal douches.

MENOPAUSE (Disorders of)
>   Single seed hawthorn (blossom)   *one handful*
>   Mistletoe (leaves and stems. Should be picked before berries
>   appear)   *one handful*
>   Sage (leaves)   *one handful*

Vaginal douches.
Hand-baths.

METRITIS:
>   Garlic   *one crushed head*
>   Single seed hawthorn (crushed blossoms)   *one handful*
>   Greater celandine (leaves and stems, semi-fresh if possible)
>   *one handful*
>   Round-leaved mallow (flowers)   *one handful*
>   Blackberry brambles (leaves)   *one handful*
>   Sage (flowers and leaves)   *one handful*

Vaginal douches.
Foot- and hand-baths.

METRORRHAGIA:

> Shepherd's purse (flowers and leaves)   *one handful*
> Milk-thistle (roots and leaves)   *one handful*
> Greater celandine (leaves and stems, semi-fresh if possible)   *one handful*
> Nettle (leaves, fresh if possible)   *one handful*
> Field horsetail (leaves)   *one handful*

Vaginal douches.

PAINFUL PERIODS:

> Milfoil (flowers)   *one handful*
> Single seed hawthorn (blossom)   *one handful*
> Shepherd's purse (whole plant)   *one handful*
> Nettle (leaves)   *one handful*
> Parsley (fresh leaves)   *one handful*
> Sage (leaves)   *one handful*

Vaginal douches.

Foot- and hand-baths.

STERILITY:

> Greater celandine (leaves and flowers, semi-fresh if possible)   *one handful*
> Corn (stigma)   *one handful*
> Peppermint (leaves and flowers)   *one handful*
> St. John's wort (leaves)   *one handful*
> Sage (leaves)   *one handful*
> Sweet violet (flowers)   *one handful*

Vaginal douches.

VAGINITIS:

> Couch-grass (grated roots)   *one handful*
> Corn poppy (flowers and crushed capsules)   *one handful*
> Round-leaved mallow (grated roots)   *one handful*
> Broad-leaved plantain (leaves, fresh if possible)   *one handful*
> Sweet violet (flowers)   *one handful*

Vaginal douches.

Appendix II

YOUR HEALTH IN YOUR GARDEN

My good herbs are to be found in our woodlands and countryside, but you won't usually find them all conveniently growing in the same spot. Certain regions contain a greater variety than others, and if you live in the country, you can find my entire pharmacopoeia growing almost on your doorstep, but wherever you live, if you wish to make use of medicinal plants all the year round, you can start preparing for winter in the spring. Those plants that nature doesn't provide you can grow yourself, and while the cultivated plants may be a little less effective than those that grow wild, they will nevertheless have enough virtues to be of help. If, like Candide, you are lucky enough to able to cultivate your own garden, keep a few spaces for these plants, which are generally as beautiful as they are useful.

I am not suggesting that you should play at being Mességué's apprentice, for certain plants can be noxious if wrongly used. Just because you don't actually swallow your macerations is no reason for assuming that they are harmless. Osmosis can be just as dangerous as any other kind of treatment.

The plants I recommend that you grow are:

ARTICHOKE	MARSH-MALLOW
BORAGE	MEADOW-SWEET
CABBAGE	MILFOIL
COMMON BROOM	ONION
DANDELION	PARSLEY
SWEET BRIER	PEPPERMINT
GARLIC	CORN POPPY
GREAT BURDOCK	CABBAGE ROSE
SINGLE SEED HAWTHORN	SAGE
SPRING HEATH	SUCCORY (CHICORY)
KNAPWEED	THYME
LAVENDER	SWEET VIOLET
MALE FERN	ROMAN CAMOMILE
ROUND-LEAVED MALLOW	

Prepare the soil carefully, using no chemical fertilizers, of course. You must also never use insecticides, pesticides, defoliating sprays; otherwise you'll be doing more harm than good.

HOW TO GROW THEM

Signs: ○ full sun   ◑ sun and shade   ● shade

ARTICHOKE (tender perennial) ◑

Even without a vegetable garden as such, you can grow one or two heads. The leaves are very beautiful and decorative. It thrives in a cool spot but hates the damp. Its favorite fertilizer is cow dung.

Buy your heads from a horticulturist, plant them fairly deep, and in autumn, earth them up high to protect them from the cold. They freeze at minus fourteen degrees Fahrenheit.

Gathering: Pick the leaves throughout the summer before the plant opens its flower, and dry them.

BORAGE (annual) ◑

It is a good-tempered, adaptable plant. Broadcast the seed in April or May in well-loosened soil. Thin out approximately 2 weeks after the shoots appear, allowing 1 foot (30 cm) between them.

Gathering: The whole plant should be picked just before flowering, and dried.

CABBAGE (annual) ◑

The symbol of peasant cooking, and a very valuable plant in phytotherapy.

If you have none in your vegetable garden and do not want to run the risk of using cabbage that has been forced with the help of chemical fertilizers, those who live in climates with mild winters can sow them in a forcing frame at the end of August. Thin out, picking the strongest and planting them deep in light soil. Earth up in mid-February to mid-March, and pick. In cold winter climates, time your planting to avoid the hot summer months—plant in either early spring or mid-summer for late autumn and early winter harvests.

If you wish to have cabbage all year round, there are different varieties that can take over one after the other.

COMMON BROOM (perennial) ○

There is only one kind of soil it dislikes: chalky soil. Sow the seed in spring on well-loosened, sifted soil. Plant the best shoots as soon as they are strong enough. They need no particular care.

Gathering: Choose the young twigs and flowers just before they reach full blossom. Dry in the shade.

DANDELION (perennial) ○ ◑ ●

Needs a moist soil in summer, but is otherwise a hardy and adaptable little plant. Sow in one or two rows, and hoe frequently. Leave them in the earth for two or three years so that the roots will gain sufficient strength.

Gathering: Pull up the roots in the spring before the plant sets its flower, or in the autumn once the above-ground portion has died back.

SWEET BRIER (perennial) ○

This is the wild rose of our countryside. In winter, dig up the suckers growing around the old plants, getting as much root as you can, and replant them, cutting them back as you would any rose bush, pruning the roots with shears and immersing them in soil and water. They do not seem to mind what kind of soil they have. Earth them up lightly. Cut back at the same time as garden roses.

Gathering: First pick the rose buds, then, after the early autumn frosts, pick the fruit, or hips, as they are commonly called.

GARLIC (annual) ○

Belongs in the vegetable garden if you have one. Plant the cloves in early autumn at a depth of 1⅕ inches (3 cm) and 5 inches (12 cm) apart. Cut them back two or three weeks before picking. They are ready to harvest the following autumn.

Warning: Garlic does not like freshly manured soil. Manure six months before.

Gathering: Clean the heads and hang them up to dry.

GREAT BURDOCK (biennial) ○

Requires no special care, prefers well-manured, light soil. The seeds cannot be bought, but are to be found anywhere in the countryside. Gather them yourself and sow them in September or early spring, dropping 4 or 5 seeds into holes about 2 inches deep and 10 inches apart. Hoe and weed as usual.

Warning: Great burdock spreads like nettles. Cut off the tips of stems before maturity.

Gathering: Roots should be harvested in the autumn of their first year or the spring of their second year. The leaves are best when picked in the spring and early summer.

SINGLE SEED HAWTHORN (perennial bush) ○

Will grow anywhere and in any kind of soil, but its chosen land is Normandy. Its blossoms are commonly called May, and whether growing as a hedge or a tree, it is always a pretty sight. Like other bushes of its kind, it requires no particular care.

If you have the patience, you can plant the whole fruit at the end of autumn, but they grow very slowly and you have to wait over two years for results.

Medicinally, their white blossoms are preferable to roses.

Gathering: Whether in the countryside or in your own garden, pick the blossom while it is still in bud and dry it.

SPRING HEATH (perennial) ○ ◑

It needs a sandy soil with plenty of leaf mold and peat moss. It likes stony and well-ventilated soil, and cannot live in heavy ground.

Sow the seeds in spring and thin out the shoots. It is, of course, quicker to uproot an entire plant growing wild, along with a big clod of earth, and replant it. It is as well to move several at once, for they will not all "take."

Gathering: Pick the flowers as soon as they start to bloom.

KNAPWEED (perennial) ◑

Likes a moist, deep, light soil. Lighten your soil with peat moss.

Seeds can be sown in early March, under a frame, or at the end of March in the open. Fifteen days after the shoots have appeared, thin and replant two feet apart. Hoe and water if it is a dry summer.

Gathering: Pull up the plants every three years and dry the roots.

LAVENDER (perennial) ○

They say it thrives only in the south of France, but this is not so. Lavender will grow anywhere, and although it might have less strength and goodness, it is still useful. It prefers dry, chalky soil.

Buy your plants from a local horticulturist, which will ensure that they are already acclimatized. They require no particular care. When they have finished flowering, cut them back pretty severely, in a dome shape.

Gathering: The flowers are picked in mid-summer as soon as they are in bloom. They dry easily.

MALE FERN (perennial) ◑ ●

This plant, with its crook like a bishop's crook, likes light and fairly damp soil with a northerly exposure. Do not hesitate to mix your soil with sand to lighten it. A hardy plant that requires no care. Because this plant is on many threatened species lists in the United States, do not gather rhizomes from wild plants. Instead, purchase your root stock from a reputed nursery.

Gathering: Break off the rhizomes in autumn and dry them.

ROUND-LEAVED MALLOW (perennial) ○

Will grow in any soil, but prefers ground rich in nitrate. Sow into seed holes in the spring, although it will give no flowers until the following year. If you need quicker results, transplant wild plants in the spring or autumn and let them grow at their own pace.

Gathering: The leaves are picked just before the plant comes into flower. From June to August you can pick the flowers and dry them very quickly, so they won't deteriorate, in a dry spot in the shade. In autumn you can take up the roots and dry them.

MARSH-MALLOW (perennial) ○

Grows best if the soil is rich, moist and light.

Sow in spring, and in due course thin and transplant. It is better to take a fragment of root stock from wild plants in autumn. You will find this by exposing the roots. Cut off the root fragments where young growth is apparent, and preserve them all winter in sand. Put them in the earth when the ground thaws.

Gathering: Pick off the young roots every year. After three years the mother root becomes woody and loses much of its goodness.

MEADOW-SWEET (perennial) ◑ ●

Will grow in any soil providing it is damp. Take root stock or young plants in autumn and replant in your garden.

Gathering: Pick the flowers at the start of the flowering season, in mid- to late summer. Hang them heads down from the rafters in the loft to dry.

MILFOIL (YARROW) (perennial) ○

Needs no special corner of its own. Can be sown along with lawn seed, and at first you can mow it when you mow the lawn. Let its flowers bloom in July however, and pick them, then mow as usual. If your lawn is partly in the shade, sow the milfoil only in sunny areas.

Gathering: Gather the umbellifers in July. In the autumn you can dry the whole plant, but do not tear it up by the roots.

ONION (annual) ◑

Likes light, sweet soils, and will thrive in any climate. I recommend the red onion, which is medically more effective. You can sow seed or buy onion sets, planting them in early spring.

PARSLEY (biennial) ◑

Likes earth rich in humus. Sow the seed from February to August.

Cover with earth sifted by hand to which a little sawdust has been added. It will not survive being buried. Two and a half months after sowing it will be up. Be careful to pick only the strongest leaves.

Since it is a biennial, parsley sends up its flower stalk the second year and then dies back. For successive harvests it is necessary to plant parsley every year.

Gathering: Pick the leaves until the first frosts, and the root in autumn.

PEPPERMINT (perennial) ◑

Prefers a light, fertile, friable soil, and benefits from a little moisture. It is at its best when its head is in the shade and its feet are in moist soil. Plant the root stock in autumn, preferably taking them from wild plants or buying young plants from your horticulturist. Water them well to help them get established, but after this they need no further care, being rather rapid-spreading plants.

Gathering: The leaves should preferably be picked before flowering. They can be dried easily.

CORN POPPY (annual) ○

To me the poppy is like a gay, sturdy peasant woman in a red skirt. It will thrive anywhere providing it is in the sun and not close to garden perennials (as opposed to perennial wild plants), which will make it wilt and die. Its own predilection for fields under cultivation indicates that it likes ground that is regularly turned over. Broadcast the seed, as nature would, in autumn or spring. Thin out in order to get finer capsules.

Gathering: From May onwards you can gather the petals, which should be dried in a dry, shady spot. Turn them frequently to prevent their turning black. Later in the year gather the capsules, when they are very ripe and already practically dry, choosing the biggest ones.

CABBAGE ROSE (perennial) ○

For the queen of flowers, choose my favorite: the rose of Provins. It likes chalky soils, and will grow happily as a climber on the house wall or as a hedge. It also looks good in clumps.

Plant like all roses, first lightening the soil, trimming the roots with pruning shears and cutting back to within one or two buds of the base. Spread out the roots and plant firmly.

Gathering: The flowers should be picked when they are buds. When they are dry, separate the petals and store.

SAGE (perennial) ○

Loses many of its qualities away from the Mediterranean climate. Likes dry, light, chalky, stony soils. Will wither in the damp. Buy young plants from your horticulturist and transplant with a little organic dress-ing. Hoe frequently. Protect with straw the first winter, as when young it can be attacked by frost.

Gathering: Flowers and leaves are picked in mid-summer. They dry easily.

SUCCORY (CHICORY) (perennial) ○ ◑

Will grow anywhere, but prefers a light, moist soil. Sow in rows in early spring. Thin out once every two weeks, leaving 6–8 inches be-tween each plant. Hoe frequently.

Gathering: Threefold. The plant should be picked after flowering; follow with the second picking in June and the third in early autumn. Pull up the roots and dry them.

THYME (tender perennial) ○

Like sage, it loses its qualities away from its native soil.

Proceed as for sage. In colder climates, mulch the plant in autumn for protection from winter frost.

SWEET VIOLET (perennial) ◑ ●

Uproot wild violet plants in the spring and replant them in your garden. It likes light, moist soil, fairly rich in plant mold, like the soil of its native woodland undergrowth. It reproduces itself by sending out run-ners. A humble little plant that can nevertheless spread far.

Gathering: As spring approaches, pick the flowers in the morning before they have seen the sun, and dry them. The leaves can be picked throughout the summer and the roots are pulled up in the autumn.

ROMAN CAMOMILE (perennial) ◑

Camomile prefers soil that is light and not clay. It should be given plenty of dressing, and will benefit from gentle hoeing. Take root stock from wild plants in early autumn and replant.

Gathering: Pick the flower (the whole head) in mid-summer, before it is fully opened.

To complete your stock of herbs, you can pick the following plants which gardeners consider as weeds:

> *In your garden:*
> — Couch-grass
> — Broad-leaved plantain
> — Shepherd's purse

Against your house:
- Greater celandine
- Nettle

When out walking:
- Buttercup
- Cow-parsnip
- Ground-ivy
- Field horsetail
- Knot-grass

Make the most of our good herbs. Picking them, in your garden or in the countryside, will be good for you, and is an easy step to good health.

Our parents and grandparents, who were closer to nature than we are, used to eat according to the season of the year. In their day you couldn't buy Cape strawberries or Dutch hothouse tomatoes in mid-winter. Clearly, a well-balanced diet should reflect the difference in the seasons, just as our calorie expenditure and need for vitamins varies throughout the year. Our body cries out for the foods that correspond to its changing needs, and it is up to us to satisfy these needs.

In the spring you must help your body to rid itself of the impurities accumulated during the winter and to renew itself. Eat more raw vegetables and greens, and instead of meat cooked in rich sauces, stick to plain grilled meat, especially spring lamb, free-range chicken and river fish. You will benefit greatly from all the fruit available at this time of the year.

To help purify your blood and your whole system, start the day by drinking a glass of vegetable juice or eating fresh fruit, lettuce, celery, apples. Lunch should be light but sustaining, whole-rye bread and yoghurt. I am never in favor of milky coffee, but even if you love it, drink tea instead, until autumn. It will be better for the state of your liver, which has been overworked by all the rich foods you ate in winter.

Start each meal with one of the raw vegetables in season—young artichoke, radishes, celery— rather than the winter vegetables: carrots, etc. Follow it with grilled meat or fish and steamed greens, which you should cook as briefly as possible. Overcooking causes vegetables to lose much of their goodness. Eat salads of dandelion and young lettuce, and whatever fruit is in season. Compensate for the lack of fruit available in early spring with milk products.

Your evening meal is the time for spring vegetable soups, fish, boiled eggs and the first fresh fruits, stewed, which should be rapidly and briefly cooked. Overstewed foods are the enemy of your figure as well as your health.

Parsley, fresh onions, cheeses, black olives and the odd handful of dried fruits will build up your defenses against colds, for don't forget the old saying; "Ne'er cast a clout till May is out." Eat "lightly" but don't waste your reserves, you'll still need them.

When summer comes you will naturally tend to choose cold meals, to drink a lot and eat too many raw vegetables. Be warned, do not eat too many tomatoes or lemons, which are known for their demineralizing effect. You must be particularly careful if you go in for a lot of sports and prolonged sun-bathing, for you run the risk of decalcification. This is the danger of summer. Compensate for it by eating celery and Camembert cheese. Don't eat the heavy meals you do in winter; drink plenty of liquids, for you are being dehydrated more, but do not touch iced fizzy drinks, however pleasant they may be.

Summer is the season when fruits and vegetables are at their best, full of natural sunshine. Make the most of them, but do not completely substitute them for your usual foods. Too much cellulose can cause serious stomach and intestinal troubles. Remember that any severe prolonged imbalance in your diet is always disastrous. Start your day with fresh fruit or vegetable juices: cucumber, celery, apricot, grapefruit. You need vitamins to withstand the scorching rays of the sun. Instead of rye bread eat wholemeal bread, and eat yoghurt. If you spend a lot of time on the beach, eat light meals, but above all, don't go out on an empty stomach. Grilled fish with herbs or some cold meat will give you the strength you need to go swimming and running and leaping about on the beach "like a native." Some cheese and ripe fruit will tide you over till evening, and remember that strawberries, if they agree with you, are good for almost everything, that cherries remineralize and cleanse the blood, that apricots are good for anemia, that pears are diuretic and peaches are laxative.

Once the really hot season is over, return to more hearty meals of grilled meat or fish with herbs, fresh tuna, chicken salad. When you eat cold meals, let it be at lunchtime, but be sure they are not icy cold, and eat a hot meal in the evening. Avoid rich stews and sauces, and if you are by the sea, make the most of the shell fish and even crustaceans, for they contain anything you might be lacking. Eat plenty of garlic and onion, and in the evening try to eat stewed fruit which, provided it has been only briefly cooked and slightly sweetened, will retain most of its active qualities, while not being tiring to your liver and intestines. Contrary to common practice, eat melon in the evening rather than at lunchtime, and do not eat it ice cold. During the holidays, one goes to bed late, walking or dancing after dinner, and melon is easily digested, especially if one is happy.

Be careful about drinks, for they are your enemy in hot weather. You will tend to drink anything that comes to hand, providing it's cold and there's plenty of it. Drink as much as you fancy, especially between meals, but not too close to eating fruit and raw vegetables, when liquid will cause distension and flatulence. Be wary of alcohol; it is an enemy of your liver and your figure. Choose instead drinks based on fresh mint, which are not only delicious but soothing and diuretic and good for the stomach.

In the autumn far-sighted animals, such as hedgehogs, dormice and squirrels, start laying up supplies for the winter. Do as they do—start to increase your daily intake of calories, calcium and phosphorus. This is also the ideal time to take a grape cure, which will prepare your system for the shocks winter has in store.

Begin the day by drinking grape juice, and start putting butter on your wholemeal bread and eating more mountain honey. Lunch can be a richer meal. Salads can give way a little to rice, preferably unpolished. This is the best season for cereals, fresh nuts, cubes of Gruyère cheese mixed with chicory and apple. Rabbits and well-fed chickens are good to eat, either grilled or roasted, and if you're tempted to eat some game, be sure it is not hung or prepared in rich sauce. Don't forget about ratatouilles, rich with olive oil and fragrant with the herbs of Provence, and choose mountain cheeses, especially if they are made locally. Grapes are still the best possible dessert.

Your evening meal, especially towards the end of autumn, should begin with beef bouillon or a vegetable soup like minestrone. Follow it with eggs or fish, and make the most of mushrooms, which are now at their best. Eat chestnuts too, cooked in milk, for they are a complete food in themselves. End your dinner with a bunch of grapes.

Your winter diet should take into account the climate you live in. The colder it is, the more calories you will expend and the more extra vitamins you will require.

You should drink plenty of orange juice, for this is the time of year to reinforce your natural defenses against colds and flu by stepping up your intake of vitamin C. Your breakfast should be more substantial, including perhaps a little mild cheese, and egg, and buttered whole-rye bread, which has laxative properties that will help you eliminate the toxins of a richer diet. Continue to eat plenty of honey.

Start your lunch with raw winter vegetables: grated carrots, red or green cabbage, celeriac, beetroot. Eat as much shell fish as you like, for the high iodine content will safeguard you in wintry weather. From time to time substitute a pot-au-feu or a succulent stew or a boiled fowl for your grilled beef or lamb. Don't forget cod, which is rich in calcium and reputedly anti-carcinogenic. Eat plenty of watercress and, providing it agrees with you, lightly cooked cabbage.

This is also the one time in the year when you can indulge in a little bacon, pork, *confit* (preserved goose) and *foie gras.*

For your evening meal you can enjoy country soups, clear meat soups, gratinées, casseroles. Winter is not the time to neglect vitamins, so eat a reasonable amount of starchy foods and salad, as well as home-made compotes and jams.

Make sure you are getting extra calcium by eating cheese of any kind, and phosphorus from brains and fish. Apples are full of goodness, but remember the old saying about oranges: "Oranges are gold in the morning, silver at noon and lead at night." Don't drink too much tea or coffee, and never touch hot toddy, but rather, mulled wine. A glass of vintage wine with your meals will help you to endure the hardships of winter.

With your system well protected by the food you eat, you need only wait for spring to start on the pleasant cycle of the seasons once again.